ZUR GESCHICHTE DER
OTO-RHINO-LARYNGOLOGIE
IN ÖSTERREICH

Eduard H. Majer / Manfred Skopec

ZUR GESCHICHTE DER OTO-RHINO-LARYNGOLOGIE IN ÖSTERREICH
HISTORY OF OTO-RHINO-LARYNGOLOGY IN AUSTRIA

Eine Text-Bild-Dokumentation
An Illustrated Documentation

Mit 127 Abbildungen

Verlag Christian Brandstätter · Wien–München

Die Abbildungen auf dem Schutzumschlag zeigen: Das Allgemeine Krankenhaus in Wien, kolorierter Kupferstich von Jos. u. Peter Schaffer, Wien Ende 18. Jh. (oben). Ludwig Türck, Gemälde von Josef Neugebauer, 1876; im Besitz der I. HNO-Klinik in Wien (links unten). Adam Politzer, unsigniertes Ölgemälde, 1887 (rechts unten).

1. Auflage

Die Bildauswahl und die graphische Gestaltung stammen von Christian Brandstätter und Franz Hanns. Die technische Betreuung erfolgte durch Franz Hanns. Die lektoratsmäßige Betreuung sowie die Übersetzung ins Englische besorgten Margaret Russell-Skopec und Manfred Skopec.

Alle Bildunterlagen stammen aus dem Besitz von E. H. Majer oder aus dem Institut für Geschichte der Medizin der Universität Wien, sofern nicht im Bildtext anders vermerkt.

Dieses Buch wurde beim Wiener Verlag in Himberg gedruckt und gebunden. Die Reproduktion der Abbildungen erfolgte bei Beissner & Co. in Wien, gesetzt wurde in der Garamond, 10 auf 10 Punkt, in der RSB Fotosatz Gesellschaft m. b. H. in Wien.

Alle Rechte, auch die des auszugsweisen Abdrucks oder der Reproduktion einer Abbildung, sind vorbehalten.
Copyright © 1985 by Christian Brandstätter Verlag & Edition, Wien
ISBN 3-85447-153-x

Christian Brandstätter Verlag & Edition Gesellschaft m. b. H. & Co KG
A-1080 Wien, Wickenburggasse 26, Telephon (0222) 48 38 14-15

INHALT/TABLE OF CONTENTS

E. H. Majer
Vorwort/Preface
7

Einleitung/Introduction
8

Die Otologen/The Otologists
11

Die Laryngologen und die Rhinologen/
The Laryngologists and Rhinologists
53

Anmerkungen/References
94

E. H. Majer
Die Vorstände der Universitätskliniken in Wien,
Graz und Innsbruck und die Abteilungsvorstände
der Allgemeinen Poliklinik in Wien/
The Heads of the University Clinics in Vienna,
Graz and Innsbruck. The Heads of Departments
of the General Policlinic in Vienna
101

E. H. MAJER
VORWORT
PREFACE

Seit der Gründung der Wiener Ohrenklinik 1873 unter Adam POLITZER und Josef GRUBER und der Laryngologischen Klinik 1870 unter Leopold SCHRÖTTER VON KRISTELLI sind gewaltige Fortschritte in der Grundlagenforschung und der Therapie der Hals-, Nasen- und Ohrenkrankheiten erzielt worden. Trotzdem ist es für jeden Arzt interessant und mitunter auch lehrreich, die Anfänge und die Entwicklung des Faches kennenzulernen.

Das Interesse an der Geschichte der Hals-, Nasen- und Ohrenheilkunde nimmt ständig zu. So erschien 1949 von R. Scott STEVENSON und Douglas GUTHRIE „A History of Oto-Laryngology", 1980 von Yves GUERRIER und Pierre MOUNIER-KUHN „Histoire des maladies de l'oreille, du nez et de la gorge", 1981 von J. WILLEMOT et al. „Naissance et développement de l'Oto-rhino-laryngologie dans l'histoire de la médecine" als Supplementband der ‚Acta Oto-Rhino-Laryngologica Belgica', 1967 eine Neuauflage von POLITZERS „Geschichte der Ohrenheilkunde" in Hildesheim, der 1980 eine Übersetzung des 1. Bandes ins Englische durch Stanley MILSTEIN, Collice PORTNOFF und Antje COLEMAN in Phoenix, Arizona, folgte.

Meine Fachausbildung für Hals-, Nasen- und Ohrenheilkunde erhielt ich an der Wiener Ohrenklinik bei Heinrich NEUMANN, dem bekannten Politzer-Schüler. Von Adam POLITZER wurde nach seiner Emeritierung 1907 der erste Band seiner „Geschichte der Ohrenheilkunde" veröffentlicht, in der er die Entwicklung des Faches von den ersten Anfängen bis zur Mitte des 19. Jahrhunderts behandelt. Im Jahr 1913 erschien der zweite Band, in dem POLITZER den Stand der Ohrenheilkunde seit 1850 in den einzelnen Ländern, darunter auch in Österreich, beschreibt. Seit der Übernahme der Leitung der HNO-Abteilung der Wiener Poliklinik 1946 mußte ich immer wieder als Sekretär unserer Fachgesellschaft, als zeitweiliger Vizepräsident bzw. Präsident zu den verschiedensten Anlässen biographisches Material für Würdigungen und Festansprachen über prominente Kliniker und Ärzte sammeln. Dabei wurde mein medizinhistorisches Interesse tatkräftigst von Erna LESKY, dem Vorstand des Instituts für Geschichte der Medizin in Wien, später von ihrem Nachfolger, Helmut WYKLICKY, unterstützt. Seit Jahren hatte ich die Absicht, aus diesen einzelnen Biographien eine kurze Geschichte unseres ganzen Faches zur Ergänzung und im Anschluß an POLITZERS „Geschichte der Ohrenheilkunde" zu verfassen. Erst durch die intensive Zusammenarbeit mit Manfred SKOPEC war dies möglich.

Ein unmittelbarer Anlaß für das Erscheinen des vorliegenden Buches im Jahr 1985 ist der 150. Geburtstag von Adam POLITZER und der aus diesem Anlaß veranstaltete gemeinsame Kongreß der Internationalen Politzergesellschaft und unserer Österreichischen Fachgesellschaft.

Dem Verlag Christian BRANDSTÄTTER gilt unser Dank für die hervorragende Ausstattung und die gelungene Dokumentation.

Since the founding of the Vienna Clinic of Otology in 1873 under Adam POLITZER and Josef GRUBER and since the establishment of the Clinic of Laryngology in 1870 under Leopold SCHRÖTTER VON KRISTELLI, giant steps have been made in the progress of research and therapy concerning diseases of the ear, nose and throat. Nevertheless it is interesting and sometimes even instructive for today's physician to become acquainted with the beginning and the development of this discipline.

Interest in the history of oto-rhino-laryngology is constantly growing. In 1949 R. Scott STEVENSON and Douglas GUTHRIE published "A History of Oto-Laryngology", followed by "Histoire des maladies de l'oreille, du nez et de la gorge" written by Yves GUERRIER and Pierre MOUNIER-KUHN in 1980. In 1981 J. WILLEMOT et al. published "Naissance et développement de l'Oto-rhino-laryngologie dans l'histoire de la médecine" as a supplemental volume to the 'Acta Oto-Rhino-Laryngologica Belgica'.

A new edition of POLITZER's "History of Otology" appeared in 1967 in Hildesheim; a translation of the first volume into English by Stanley MILSTEIN, Collice PORTNOFF and Antje COLEMAN was published in Phoenix, Arizona, in 1980.

I received my special training in oto-rhino-laryngology at the Vienna Clinic of Otology under Heinrich NEUMANN, the reputable student of POLITZER. After Adam POLITZER became professor emeritus in 1907 the first volume of his "History of Otology" was published, in which he deals with the development of the discipline from its beginning to the mid-19th century. In 1913 the second volume appeared, in which POLITZER described the status of otology since 1850 in various countries, Austria among them. Since I became head of the ENT department of the Vienna Policlinic I have repeatedly had to gather biographical material on prominent clinicians and physicians to be presented at various occasions in my function as secretary, acting vice-president, and president of our society. In the process my interest in medical history has been energetically supported by Erna LESKY, former Head of the Institute for the History of Medicine in Vienna and later by her successor, Helmut WYKLICKY. For years I have had the intention of drawing these brief biographical sketches together to make a short history of our discipline as a complement and supplement to POLITZER's "History of Otology". The realization of this project has only become possible through intensive collaboration with Manfred SKOPEC.

The immediate occasion for the publication of this book in 1985 is the 150th birthday of Adam POLITZER and the resulting joint congress of the International Politzer Society and our Austrian Society for ENT, Head- and Neck-Surgery. We thank the publisher Christian BRANDSTÄTTER for the outstanding layout and the effective documentation.

EINLEITUNG
INTRODUCTION

Im Jahre 1883 schrieb der seit 1877 in Frankfurt am Main zunächst als „Nasen- und Hals-Arzt" und später auch als Ohrenarzt praktizierende Maximilian BRESGEN nach Studien in Wien in einer Artikelserie in der von Johann SCHNITZLER herausgegebenen und redigierten Wiener Medizinischen Presse in Hinblick auf die Bedeutung der Spezialisierung in der Medizin: „Krankheiten, welche man Jahrhunderte lang nicht als solche gekannt oder mit anderen stets verwechselt oder welche man überhaupt nicht für eine Krankheit oder vielleicht nur als eine ganz unbedeutende, unwesentliche angesehen hat, sind durch die Bemühungen der Spezialisten, respektive Solcher, welche sich besonders mit ihnen beschäftigt haben, richtig oder richtiger bewerthet worden . . . Zu welcher Höhe hat sich nicht die Augenheilkunde entwickelt! Und welche Fortschritte hat nicht die Ohrenheilkunde gemacht, und welche wird sie erst noch machen, nachdem wir in den jüngsten Jahren die Erkrankungen der Nasenhöhle und des Rachenraumes besser haben würdigen gelernt! Und welche grossartigen Fortschritte hat nicht unsere Kenntniss von den Krankheiten des Kehlkopfes, der Luftröhre, der Rachenhöhle und insbesondere, wie schon erwähnt, der Nasenhöhle in den letzten 25 Jahren erfahren! . . . Ich will nicht erst alle Spezialitäten der Medizin besonders durchgehen; es genügt, zu sagen und zu wissen, dass in allen grossartige Fortschritte, und zwar gerade durch Arbeitsheilung, erzielt worden sind."[1] BRESGEN schloß aber seine diesbezügliche Artikelserie mit einem „Ruf nach Sammlung": „Wie ich schon . . . eingehend dargelegt habe, ist der Ruf nach Sammlung in der Medicin ein wohlberechtigter. Ich habe aber auch erwiesen, dass eine Trennung der Medicin in einzelne Specialfächer in Folge der Erweiterung unseres Wissens im Allgemeinen und zur Bewältigung der immensen Casuistik nothwendig erfolgen musste . . . Als besonders berechtigt musste sich . . . bei meiner Untersuchung ergeben, dass ein Lehrstuhl für Rhino-Laryngologie . . . errichtet werden müsse. Ich legte auch dar, dass diesem Specialfache die gleiche Berechtigung wie der Ophthalmologie und gar der Otologie zur Seite stehe. Von der ersteren zeigte ich früher schon, dass sie in sehr vielen Fällen ohne die Rhinologie nicht zu befriedigenden Resultaten zu gelangen vermag . . . In der Praxis wird sich die Verschmelzung der Otologie mit der Rhino-Laryngologie überraschend schnell vollziehen. Denn immer mehr bricht sich die Ueberzeugung Bahn, dass die Rhino-Pharyngologie für die Otologie und Laryngologie nahezu von gleicher Bedeutung ist und diese beiden ohne Rhinologie keine wirklichen und dauernden Erfolge zu erringen vermögen."[2]
Bis heute läßt die Benennung des Specialfaches den heterogenen Ursprung der darinnen zusammengefaßten Disziplinen erkennen. Wie Hans-Heinz EULNER in seiner umfassenden Darstellung der Entwicklung der medizinischen Spezialfächer an den Universitäten des deutschen Sprachgebietes aufzeigt,[3] sind die genannten Disziplinen nicht so sehr durch innere Notwendigkeit, als durch äußere Zweckmäßigkeit zusammengeführt worden. War die Otologie zunächst mehr ein

Maximilian BRESGEN wrote a series of articles in 1883 in regard to the importance of specialization in medicine. BRESGEN had studied in Vienna among other cities, and since 1877 he had practiced in Frankfurt am Main, first as a "Throat-and-Nose-Doctor", then as an ear-specialist. His articles appeared in the 'Wiener Medizinische Presse', published and edited by Johann SCHNITZLER: "Diseases which for years have gone unrecognized or were mistaken for other maladies, or which were not regarded as diseases at all, or if so, only insignificant, unessential ones, have become more accurately assessed through the efforts of specialists, or those who have been particularly associated with these diseases. . . . What heights has ophthalmology not reached! And what progress has ophthalmology not made and will continue to make, now that we have plunged the depths of knowledge concerning diseases of the nasal and pharyngeal cavities in the most recent years! And what magnificent progress our knowledge of the diseases of the larynx, trachea, pharynx, and particularly the nasal cavity has made in the past 25 years! And how our conception of the importance of the nasal cavity and the diseases thereof has changed so completely in recent years, such that we are now just beginning to realize how important this little organ is for the entire organism. . . . I do not want to enumerate all the special fields of medicine; suffice it to say and to know that in each one of them, gigantic progress has been made through division of work."[1]
BRESGEN, however, closed his series of articles with a "call for unity": "As I have clearly shown, I am well justified in calling for a unity of medical knowledge. I have also proven, however, that a division in the various special medical disciplines was necessary as a result of our expanding knowledge in general and to cope with the enormous number of cases. . . . My studies have further shown that the establishment of a chair for Rhino-Laryngology is particularly justifiable. I have proven that this special field is just as legitimate as ophthalmology or otology. I have shown that regarding otology, many cases can not achieve sufficient results without the knowledge of rhinology. In practice the fusion of otology and rhino-laryngology will take place surprisingly fast. For more and more physicians are convinced that rhino-pharyngology is of almost equal importance to otology as to laryngology, and that both of the latter are incapable of achieving real and lasting results without rhinology."[2]
Even today the heterogeneous origin of this discipline can be surmised from the compound name given to it. As the medico-historian Hans-Heinz EULNER points out in his detailed portrayal of the development of the special fields of medicine at the universities in German-speaking countries[3], the disciplines cited came together not so much by nature of inherent necessity as by external expediency. While otology was primarily a branch of surgery, laryngology developed primarily as a sub-field of internal medicine. Rhinology was continually regarded by both disciplines as "belonging to it" on the grounds of its close connections to either field. In 1962

Zweig der Chirurgie, entwickelte sich die Laryngologie vor allem aus der inneren Medizin heraus. Die Rhinologie wurde stets von den beiden Disziplinen auf Grund ihrer Beziehung zur einen wie zur anderen Seite als ihnen zugehörig betrachtet. Im Jahr 1962 resümierte Joseph MATZKER in einer Arbeit zur Geschichte des Spezialfaches: „Der Oto-Rhino-Laryngologie als einem organologisch abgegrenzten Fach ist die Fürsorge für vier wichtige Sinnesorgane anvertraut: das Ohr, das Gleichgewichts-, das Geruchs- und das Geschmacksorgan. Absolut lebenswichtige Funktionskomplexe (freie Atempassage, Schluckmechanismus) sind in die Obhut vorwiegend des Otolaryngologen gegeben. Die Abrundung dieser Disziplin auf die derzeit von ihr gepflegten Arbeitsgebiete ist sinnvoll sowohl im Hinblick auf die anatomischen und patho-physiologischen Gegebenheiten als auch auf die gerade noch vorhandene Überschaubarkeit durch einen einzelnen. Zwar lassen sich in letzter Zeit – vorwiegend in Amerika – wieder Tendenzen zu weiterer Spezialisierung und damit Aufsplitterung des Faches feststellen (reine Oto-, Audio-, Laryngo-, Rhino- und Bronchologen); in Europa jedoch wird von allen maßgeblichen Fachvertretern und allen Fachkliniken die historisch gewachsene Abgrenzung der Oto-Rhino-Laryngologie als optimal angesehen und in ihrer Integrität zu erhalten getrachtet."[4] – Wem fielen hier nicht GOETHES Worte ein: „Bei Erweiterung unseres Wissens macht sich von Zeit zu Zeit eine Umdeutung nötig; sie geschieht meistens nach neueren Maximen, bleibt aber immer provisorisch."[5,6]

Wodurch kam es zur Vereinigung dieser auf den ersten Blick so heterogen scheinenden Fächer? Wohl in erster Linie durch die Möglichkeit, mit den in der zweiten Hälfte des 19. Jahrhunderts entwickelten Geräten vorher kaum sichtbar zu machende Einzelheiten in der Tiefe von Ohr, Nase und Kehlkopf direkt oder indirekt zu erkennen.[7] Obwohl man bereits in der Antike das Sonnenlicht für die direkte Beobachtung etwa des äußeren Gehörorgans heranzog,[8] dauerte es doch bis zum 19. Jahrhundert, daß Methoden entwickelt wurden, um auch die der direkten Beleuchtung unzugänglichen Körperhöhlen untersuchen zu können. Während die Laryngologie mit der Erfindung des Kehlkopfspiegels eigentlich erst beginnen konnte und dadurch als Disziplin einen „dramatischen"[9] Anfang nahm, wie später noch auszuführen sein wird, wuchs die Ohrenheilkunde allmählich auf der Grundlage detaillierter Kenntnis der normalen und pathologischen Anatomie des Ohres. Die neuen untersuchungstechnischen, anatomischen, physiologischen und pathologisch-anatomischen Grundlagen ermöglichten es einer ersten Generation mutiger und oft gegen eine noch verständnislose Umwelt ankämpfender Einzelpersönlichkeiten, die Oto-Rhinologie einerseits und die Rhino-Laryngologie andererseits als Spezialfächer zu betreiben. Welche Schwierigkeiten die Pioniere der heute vereinten Disziplin zu überwinden hatten und mit welchem Idealismus sie ihre wissenschaftlichen Leistungen vollbrachten, geht allein schon aus der Tatsache hervor, daß es in Österreich – und dies trifft natürlich nicht nur für Österreich zu – bis zum Ende des 19. Jahrhunderts keine besoldeten Universitätsprofessoren der genannten Fächer gab. Deshalb sollen diese Ärzte im Mittelpunkt unserer Betrachtung stehen. Vergessen wollen wir dabei aber nicht, daß ein Teil der berühmten Pioniere unseres Faches aus dem Bereich der alten Österreichisch-ungarischen Monarchie stammt und in die Hauptstadt des Reiches Erbgut der verschiedensten Nationen mitgebracht hat.

Joseph MATZKER summarized the development in a paper on the history of the special field: "The care of four vital sense organs is entrusted to oto-rhino-laryngology: the ear, the organs of balance, of smell, and of taste. Absolutely vital functional complexes (non-constructed breathing passage, swallowing mechanism) have been more or less assigned to the oto-laryngologist. The rounding off of this discipline into the divisions as practiced today is sensible in regard to both the anatomical and patho-physiological factors and in regard to the fact that the field can just be mastered in all its dimensions by a single person. Recently – particularly in America – the trend has been towards further specialization and thereby a splintering of the field (pure otologists, audiologists, laryngologists, rhinologists and bronchologists). But in Europe, at least, the historically inherent development of oto-rhino-laryngology is seen by all leading representatives and clinics of the discipline to be optimal and therefore worth being maintained."[4] Who would not think of GOETHE's words here: "When expanding our knowledge, a form of rethinking is necessary from time to time; it mostly is done according to newer maxims, but it always remains temporary."[5,6]

How did this union of – at first sight – such differing disciplines come about? Primarily through the possibility of making the details in the depths of the ear, nose and larynx directly or indirectly recognizable through the use of instruments which had not been invented until the second half of the 19th century.[7] Although sunlight was used already in ancient times to directly observe the outer ear[8], it was not until the 19th century that methods were developed to examine cavities which could not be reached by direct illumination. While laryngology had its origin in the invention of the laryngoscope – giving it a "dramatic" entrance as a discipline, as will be described later – otology grew gradually upon the foundation of detailed knowledge of the normal and pathological anatomy of the ear. New technical, anatomical, physiological and pathological-anatomical groundwork made it possible for a new generation of courageous individuals, who often had to struggle against yet unappreciative colleagues, to further oto-rhinology on the one hand and rhino-laryngology on the other hand as special disciplines. What difficulties the pioneers of this joint discipline had to overcome, and with what idealism they attained their scientific achievements can be seen in the fact that there were no salaried professors teaching these subjects in Austria at the universities until the end of the 19th century – and Austria is by no means an exception. For this reason these physicians will be the focus of our attention. We do not want to forget, though, that some of the famous pioneers of our discipline came from the regions of the old Austro-Hungarian Empire and brought with them an inheritance from the most various of nations.

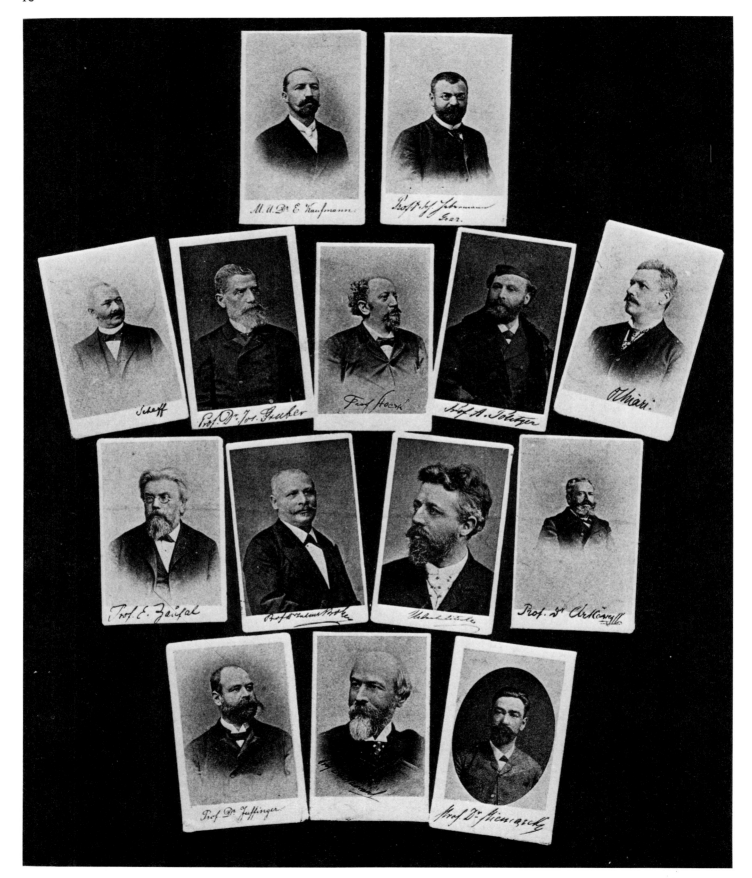

DIE OTOLOGEN
THE OTOLOGISTS

Als Adam POLITZER (1835–1920) am 1. Oktober 1907 von der Wiener Universitäts-Ohrenklinik schied, sagte er bei der Abschiedsfeier: „Mit dem heutigen Tage schließt der erste historische Abschnitt der Otiatrie an unserer Universität ab."[10] Erna LESKY spricht in diesem Zusammenhang von einem Epochenbewußtsein des ‚grand old man' in der Alser Straße für sein Fach.[11] In Anbetracht der Leistungen POLITZERS für die Ohrenheilkunde – seine wissenschaftliche und didaktische Tätigkeit umfaßt einen Zeitraum von einem halben Jahrhundert, und es gibt kein Gebiet des Spezialfaches, auf dem er nicht Grundlegendes geschaffen hätte – standen ihm solche Worte gewiß zu und klangen nicht überheblich.

Um die Mitte des 19. Jahrhunderts gab es nur zwei Ärzte in Wien, die sich mit Ohrenkrankheiten beschäftigten: Ignaz GULZ (1814–1874) und Ignaz GRUBER (1803–1872). Obzwar 1845 an der Wiener medizinischen Fakultät für Ohrenheilkunde habilitiert[12], behandelte GULZ in seiner Wiener Praxis neben Ohren- auch Augenkranke. Der Schwerpunkt seiner ärztlichen Tätigkeit verlagerte sich allmählich so sehr auf die Behandlung von Augenkrankheiten, er übte auch die Tätigkeit eines „Armenaugenarztes der Haupt- und Residenzstadt" aus, daß er schließlich als Augenarzt galt und sogar für die Besetzung der Lehrkanzel für Augenheilkunde in Wien nach dem Tode von Anton VON ROSAS (1791–1855) vom Professorenkollegium vorgeschlagen wurde.[13] Dies dürfte wohl auch die Erklärung dafür sein, wieso POLITZER für sich in Anspruch nahm, der erste Dozent für Ohrenheilkunde in Wien gewesen zu sein.[14] Die Tätigkeit von GULZ als Augen- und Ohrenarzt läßt an Ferdinand VON ARLT (1812–1887) denken, der übrigens Studiengenosse und Freund von GULZ war. ARLT schreibt: „In die Zeit meiner privatärztlichen Thätigkeit fällt auch die Bemühung, Ohrenheilkunde zu studiren und mich als Dozent dieses Faches zu habilitiren. Anfang Jänner 1844 wurde mir gestattet, Ohrenkranke auf die Abtheilungszimmer des Prof. FISCHER aufzunehmen und auch das Taubstummeninstitut zu meinen Vorträgen zu benutzen. Obwohl ich mich sehr viel mit Anfertigung anatomischer Präparate (physiologischer und pathologischer) befasst hatte, vermochte ich doch nicht, in diesem Fache etwas Erwähnenswerthes zu leisten. Dennoch freue ich mich, hier bemerken zu können, dass einer der ersten Ohrenärzte unserer Zeit, Professor v. TRÖLTSCH, seinen ersten Unterricht in diesem Fache bei mir erhalten hat, als er mich zunächst bei meinen Vorträgen über Augenheilkunde kennen gelernt hatte. Prag war die erste Universität in Oesterreich, an welcher ein besonderes Collegium über Ohrenheilkunde abgehalten wurde."[15] ARLT wandte sich bekanntlich auch ganz der Ophthalmologie zu und wurde, als er 1856 von Prag als Nachfolger ROSAS' nach Wien kam, zum Erneuerer der österreichischen Augenheilkunde.[16]

Der zweite Ohrenspezialist in Wien war damals der schon genannte Ignaz GRUBER, der Vater des Hygienikers Max GRUBER. Im Gegensatz zu GULZ spezialisierte sich GRUBER

When Adam POLITZER (1835–1920) retired from his chair at the Vienna University Clinic of Otology on October 1, 1907, he could rightly and proudly state: "Today the first historical period of otology at our university has come to an end."[10] Erna LESKY refers to "the grand old man" of the Alser Strasse as having had an epochal awareness for his field of medicine.[11] When one considers POLITZER's achievements in his field of otology – his scientific and didactic works span half a century and there is no area in his discipline in which he did not lay some foundation – such words were certainly justified and not presumptuous.

In the mid-19th century there were only two physicians in Vienna who concerned themselves with otology: Ignaz GULZ (1814–1874) and Ignaz GRUBER (1803–1872). Although GULZ was made lecturer for otology at the Vienna medical faculty in 1845,[12] he treated eye patients as well as ear patients in his Vienna practice. The focus of his medical profession gradually changed to the treatment of patients with eye diseases – he functioned as "Eye Doctor of the Indigents in the Imperial City" – so that he ultimately gained a reputation as an ophthalmologist and was even considered by the College of Professors as successor to the chair for ophthalmology in Vienna following the death of Anton von ROSAS (1791–1855).[13] This is probably also the reason why POLITZER claimed himself to have been the first *Docent* (lecturer) for otology in Vienna.[14] GULZ's activities as eye and ear doctor are reminiscent of Ferdinand von ARLT (1812–1887), who was, incidentally, a friend of GULZ'. ARLT writes: "During the time when I had my private medical practice, I also studied otology and tried to become a lecturer in this field. In the beginning of January, 1844, I was permitted to receive ear patients in the ward of Prof. FISCHER and to use the rooms of the Institute for the Deaf for my lectures. Although I had devoted much time to making anatomical models (physiological and pathological) I was never quite able to accomplish anything of significance in this discipline. Nevertheless, I am happy to mention that one of the first otologists of our time, Prof. v. TRÖLTSCH, received his first instruction in this field from me, when we became acquainted at my lectures on ophthalmology. Prague was the first university in Austria at which lectures on otology were held."[15] ARLT later dedicated himself to ophthalmology when he left Prague to become ROSAS' successor in Vienna in 1856 and became the renewer of this discipline in Austria.[16]

The second ear specialist in Vienna at that time was Ignaz GRUBER, father of the hygienist Max GRUBER. In contrast to GULZ, GRUBER specialized in the treatment of ear diseases, "so that after a short period of time not only Austrian but also German, English, and French physicians visited him at his medical practice, to be instructed by him. In scientific circles his name became known through his invention of the unsplit ear speculum (1838), which significantly improved upon the method for examining the ear, and is still used today."[17]

Neither GRUBER nor GULZ did scientific research in the field

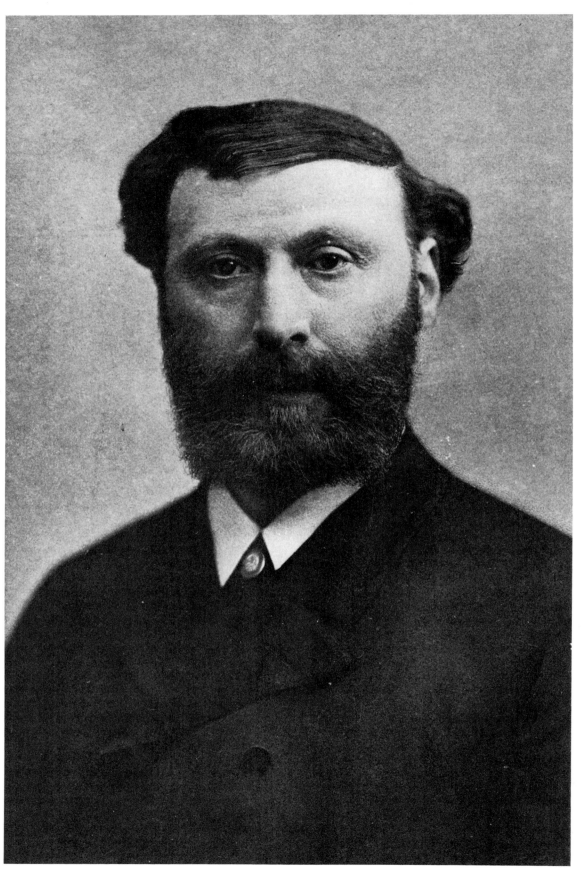

Adam Politzer. Photographie von V. Angerer, ohne Ort und Jahr.

Adam Politzer. Undated photograph by V. Angerer.

Seite 10: Die Professoren der medizinischen Fakultäten von Österreich–Ungarn um 1900.
Otiater, Laryngologen und Odontologen.
Beilage zur Wiener Medizinischen Wochenschrift (um 1900).

*Page 10: The Professors of the Medical Faculties within the Austro-Hungarian Empire around 1900.
Otologists, Laryngologists and Odontologists.
In a supplement to the "Wiener Medizinische Wochenschrift" (around 1900).*

auf die Behandlung von Ohrenkrankheiten, „so dass nach kurzer Zeit seiner Thätigkeit in dieser Richtung nicht allein inländische, sondern auch deutsche, englische und französische Aerzte seine Ordinationen besuchten, um von ihm Belehrung zu erhalten. In wissenschaftlichen Kreisen machte er durch die Erfindung seines, noch jetzt im Gebrauche stehenden ungespaltenen Ohrentrichters (1838), der die Untersuchungsmethode des Gehörorganes wesentlich verbesserte, seinen Namen allgemein geachtet."[17]
Weder I. GRUBER noch GULZ betätigten sich wissenschaftlich auf dem Gebiete der Otologie. Eine Lehrstätte für dieselbe war noch nicht gegründet; die Behandlung Ohrenkranker in den Spitälern beschränkte sich auf Ausspritzen von Ohrenschmalz, Einträufeln adstringierender Flüssigkeiten bei Ohrenfluß, Auskratzen von Fisteln am Warzenfortsatz und gelegentliche Extraktionen von Sequestern und Polypen.
In Österreich beginnt der wissenschaftliche Aufschwung der Ohrenheilkunde erst in den sechziger Jahren des vorigen Jahrhunderts, und zwar von Großbritannien ausgehend, wo unter Joseph TOYNBEE (1815–1866) in London und William Robert WILDE (1815–1876) in Dublin schon seit dem Beginn der vierziger Jahre die systematische Erforschung der Ohrenerkrankungen eingesetzt hatte.[18] TOYNBEE und WILDE forderten, daß einzig und allein in der Erweiterung und Vertiefung der Erkenntnisse in der pathologischen Anatomie ein Fortschritt in der Diagnostik, in der Beurteilung der Ohrenerkrankungen zu erwarten sei, und man ohne gründliche Kenntnis der pathologisch-anatomischen Vorgänge an eine rationelle Therapie nicht denken könne. Ebenso wie in den anderen medizinischen Disziplinen mußte auch in der Ohrenheilkunde Carl VON ROKITANSKYS (1804–1878) Leitgedanke, „... die Tathsachen vom rein anatomischen Standpunkt wissenschaftlich zu ordnen und dabei eine ihre Sonderung und Zusammenfassung fachgemäß rechtfertigende, allgemeine pathologische Anatomie zu schaffen ..." und „... zu zeigen, daß und wie die Tathsachen für die Diagnose am Lebenden zu verwerthen seien ...",[19] die Basis für den Aufbau der Diagnostik und Therapie der Ohrenerkrankungen bilden.
Wollte die Wiener Medizin auch auf dem Gebiet der Ohrenheilkunde mit dem Ausland konkurrenzfähig werden, würde es eines mit den Methoden seiner Zeit vertrauten Otologen bedürfen. Dies zu erkennen und auch die entsprechende Initiative ergriffen zu haben ist das Verdienst des Internisten Johann VON OPPOLZER (1808–1871), des Förderers der Spezialfächer, der 1861 einen eben promovierten (1859), ihm geeignet scheinenden jungen Mann auf Reisen schickte, damit er an den damals wichtigsten Stätten otiatrischen Unterrichts otologisches Wissen sammeln könne: den aus Alberti in Ungarn gebürtigen Adam POLITZER,[20] der bereits 1860 im Laboratorium Carl LUDWIGS (1835–1920) im Josephinum zwei wichtige Arbeiten verfaßt hatte: die eine über die Innervationsverhältnisse der Binnenmuskeln des Ohres, in welcher POLITZER nachwies, daß der M. tensor tympani vom Trigeminus, der M. stapedius vom Fazialis innerviert wird, und die zweite über den Einfluß der Luftdruckschwankungen in der Trommelhöhle auf die Druckverhältnisse im Labyrinth. Bei VON TRÖLTSCH in Würzburg studierte POLITZER die Klinik der Ohrenerkrankungen und die Technik der damals bereits bekannten Katheterisierung der Eustachischen Röhre. Beim Histologen KÖLLIKER in Würzburg arbeitete er sich in die mikroskopische Untersuchung des Cortischen Organs

of otology; a place for its study had not yet been founded. The treatment of ear patients in hospitals was limited to the flushing out of ear-wax, the administering of ear-drops of astringent liquids in cases of otorrhoea or otorrhagia, the scraping out of fistulas on the mastoid process, and the occasional extraction of sequestrums and polyps.
The rise of otology as a science in Austria began in the 1860s, receiving its impetus from Great Britain, where under Joseph TOYNBEE (1815–1866) in London and William Robert WILDE (1815–1876) in Dublin the systematic study of ear diseases had already commenced in the 1840s.[18] TOYNBEE and WILDE maintained that an advance in diagnosis could only be attained through a broader and deeper knowledge of pathological anatomy, and that only with an improved and thorough knowledge of the pathological-anatomical processes was a rational therapy thinkable. Just as in the other medical disciplines, the main ideas of Carl v. ROKITANSKY (1804–1878) must now also form the basis for the development of diagnosis and therapy in otology: "... sorting the facts scientifically on a purely anatomical basis and thereby creating the subject of general pathological anatomy which would justify its separate existence as such ..." and "... demonstrating the applicability of the facts and their utilization for diagnosis in live patients."[19] If the Vienna School of Medicine wanted to be able to compete with other countries in the area of otology, it would be necessary to produce an otologist who was familiar with contemporary methods in his field. To have recognized this fact and acted accordingly was the merit of the internal specialist Johann von OPPOLZER (1808–1871), a promoter of special disciplines. In 1861 he sent a young man who had recently finished his medical studies (1859) and seemed suitable to the task to the various locations at which otiatry and otology were being instructed: Adam POLITZER (1835–1920)[20] from Alberti in Hungary. In 1860 POLITZER had already demonstrated the relationships of the innervation of the m. tensor tympani and m. stapedius in animal experiments by stimulating the fifth and seventh nerves in the laboratory of the physiologist Carl LUDWIG (1835–1920) at the Josephinum in Vienna. He published a second paper on air pressure fluctuations of the middle ear influencing the pressure conditions in the labyrinth. His study trip led him to Würzburg to KÖLLIKER, where he increased his abilities with the microscope, and to Heinrich MÜLLER, where he showed the pressure equilibrium in the middle ear during swallowing in manometer studies of the external auditory canal; then to HELMHOLTZ in Heidelberg, where he received new incentives. On the basis of his experiments in Claude BERNARD's laboratory in Paris and in the acoustic institute of Rudolf KÖNIG, he demonstrated the oscillations of the auditory ossicle after tonal stimulation even before HELMHOLTZ, on which Claude BERNARD reported in the Académie des sciences. A commission was appointed to verify POLITZER's observations and findings. Two dogs had to be purchased, which POLITZER had to pay for out of his own pocket. This sum was "quite a burden to his travel account."[21] – It is possible that the invention of the telephone by Alexander Graham BELL in 1876 was stimulated by these experiments made by POLITZER. With J. TOYNBEE, the father of British otology, in London, POLITZER had the opportunity to study TOYNBEE's extensive collection of temporal bones in detail and thus became familiar with the fundamental significance of pathological anatomy and histology for correct diagnosis of disorders of the ear.[22]

ein. Im Laboratorium Heinrich MÜLLERS in Würzburg machte er auch die für die spätere Entdeckung seines nach ihm benannten Verfahrens so wichtige Beobachtung, daß der Schluckakt einen Druckausgleich zwischen Paukenhöhle und Nasenrachenraum ermöglicht.

Über Heidelberg, wo er HELMHOLTZ seine bisherigen Befunde vortrug, ging er nach Paris. Dort, im Institute MÉNIÈRES, machte er Studien über Taubstummheit und stellte im akustischen Institut Rudolf KÖNIGS seine Untersuchungen über die Fortleitung des Schalles im Gehörorgan an und wies – noch vor HELMHOLTZ – die Schwingungen der einzelnen Gehörknöchelchen bei Einwirkung von Tönen nach. Claude BERNARD berichtete darüber in der Académie des sciences, die daraufhin zur Überprüfung eine Kommission bestellte, von der die Richtigkeit der Beobachtungen POLITZERS bestätigt wurde. Allerdings mußten zwei Hunde angeschafft werden, die POLITZER aus eigener Tasche bezahlen mußte, wodurch „seine Reisekasse schwer belastet wurde"[21]. Es ist durchaus möglich, daß die Erfindung des Telephons durch Alexander Graham BELL 1876 durch POLITZERS Untersuchungen angeregt wurde.

Von Paris ging er nach London, wo er bei TOYNBEE dessen umfangreiche Sammlung pathologisch-anatomischer Ohrpräparate studieren und so die grundlegende Bedeutung der pathologischen Anatomie und Histologie für die richtige Beurteilung von Ohrenkrankheiten kennenlernen konnte.[22]

Dann kehrte POLITZER wieder nach Wien zurück. Lassen wir ihn selbst das Folgende berichten: „Als mir im Jahre 1861 durch das einstimmige Votum des Professorenkollegiums die erste Dozentur für Ohrenheilkunde an der Wiener Universität verliehen wurde, fand ich keinerlei Lehrbehelfe für das neue Spezialfach vor.

Mit inniger Dankbarkeit gedenke ich der liebevollen Förderung, die mir von meinen unvergeßlichen Lehrern ROKITANSKY, SKODA, OPPOLZER, ARLT, Karl und Gustav BRAUN und Prim. KOLISKO zuteil wurde, die mir das Material ihrer Kliniken und Abteilungen behufs wissenschaftlicher Untersuchungen überließen und denen ich es zu verdanken hatte, daß ich in verhältnismäßig kurzer Zeit über ein ansehnliches Material von Kranken und pathologisch-anatomischen Präparaten zu verfügen hatte.

Trotz des allseitigen Interesses, welches die Fakultät der neuen Disziplin entgegenbrachte, hatte die Otiatrie noch lange mit den ererbten Vorurteilen, nicht nur der großen Massen, sondern auch der praktischen Aerzte zu kämpfen. Es fehlten ihr trotz des ehrlichen Strebens und der bereits sichtbaren Erfolge jene äußerlichen Attribute, die einem Spezialfache nach außen hin ein gewisses Ansehen verleihen. In erster Reihe machte sich der Mangel passender Unterrichtsräume fühlbar. So verdanke ich es nur OPPOLZER, durch dessen Herzensgüte und Wohlwollen alle jüngeren Kräfte gefördert wurden, daß ich in einem Krankensaale seiner Klinik die Kurse abhalten konnte, während dem Dozenten Josef GRUBER ein kleiner Raum des Krankenhauses für seine Ambulanz zugewiesen wurde.

Erst 1873 wurde auf Vorschlag des Professorenkollegiums von der Unterrichtsverwaltung die Errichtung einer stationären Ohrenklinik beschlossen und zu dessen Vorständen Professor GRUBER und ich ernannt. Ich möchte hier die historische Tatsache festhalten, daß der Ruhm, die *erste otiatrische Klinik* ins Leben gerufen zu haben, unserer Fakultät unbestritten bleiben wird."[23]

Then POLITZER returned to Vienna where he reported the following: "When I became the first lecturer for otology at the University of Vienna in 1861 through the unanimous vote of the College of Professors there were no teaching aids extant for this special field. With deep gratefulness I remember the loving encouragement afforded me by my unforgettable teachers ROKITANSKY, SKODA, OPPOLZER, ARLT, Karl and Gustav BRAUN and Primarius KOLISKO. They entrusted to me material from their clinics and departments for scientific research, and it was only with their help that I had at my disposal, after a relatively short period of time, ample material concerning patients and a sizeable collection of pathological-anatomical models.

Despite the great interest which the medical faculty accorded the new discipline, otiatry had to struggle for a long time against deep-seated prejudice, not only of the masses but also of the general practitioners. In spite of all honest efforts and the already visible success of the discipline, some outward attribute which usually lends a special field respectability was missing. Foremost, the lack of suitable instruction rooms was noticeable. I am indebted to OPPOLZER – through whose goodness and encouragement we novices profited – for being able to hold classes in a ward of his department, while lecturer Josef GRUBER had to make do with a small room of the hospital for treating his patients. It was not until 1873 that the Administration, upon recommendation of the College of Professors, decided to establish a stationary Clinic of Otology, the direction of which Prof. GRUBER and I were entrusted with. I hereby wish to establish the historical fact that our faculty should be given credit for having founded the *world's first clinic of otiatry*."[23]

This clinic consisted of one large ward which could be partitioned into two rooms. Josef GRUBER (1827–1900) was in charge of the men's ward with eleven beds, and Adam POLITZER headed the women's ward with eight beds. In this small sick-room operations were performed, and the examination and treatment of an ever increasing number of out-patients were conducted. It was not until 1898 that two new rooms were added – a treatment room for out-patients and an operating room. "Never had a department been established with so little expenditure nor had such an effect been exerted on the whole world from a single room as from the department of POLITZER. The minister could rightfully state in 1894, when he proposed GRUBER and POLITZER for the title of full professors, that 'practically all lecturers in otology at the University of Vienna, as well as most professors at the universities of Germany and other countries are considered as . . . students of these two professors'."[24]

When POLITZER retired from teaching in 1907 he received from his students a valedictory address containing the signatures of 366 otologists from Europe, America, Asia, Africa, and Australia. The accompanying words say: "Nearly half a century has passed since you began your lectures on otology; . . . Those who received instruction and advice from you number in the thousands, how innumerable must be those who through your teachings have received their cure, health, and, indeed, even life! . . . Out of a small wayward, little appreciated special field otology has grown to be a recognized, outstanding, comprehensive, legitimate discipline of medicine in these forty-five years; out of a wealth of individual therapeutic and diagnostic knowledge a systematic foundation has been laid on the basis of proven anatomical-

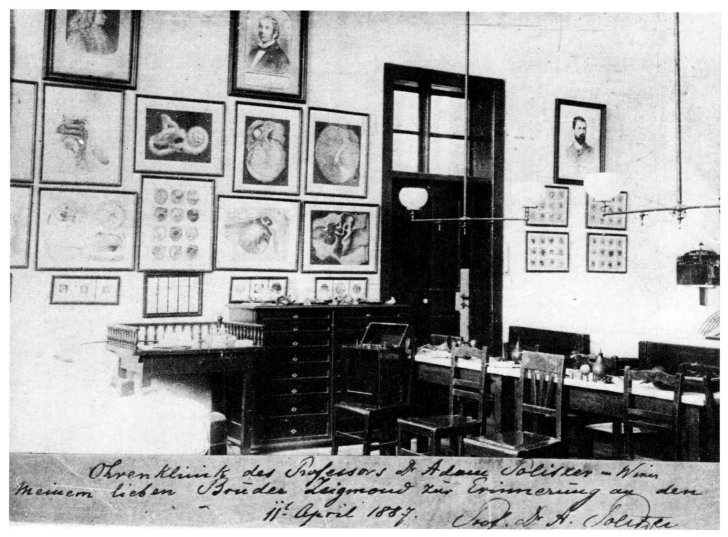

Oben: Photographie mit eigenhändiger Widmung Politzers.
Unten: Adam Politzer als Vorstand der Ohrenklinik im Allgemeinen Krankenhaus in Wien und seine Mitarbeiter. In der 1. Reihe von links nach rechts: Ruttin, Leidler, Alexander, Politzer, Neumann, Bárány, unbekannt, Frey.

Top: Photograph with dedication in Politzer's own hand.
Bottom: Adam Politzer as head of the Clinic of Otology at the Vienna General Hospital, with his staff. In the first row from left to right: Ruttin, Leidler, Alexander, Politzer, Neumann, Bárány, unknown, Frey.

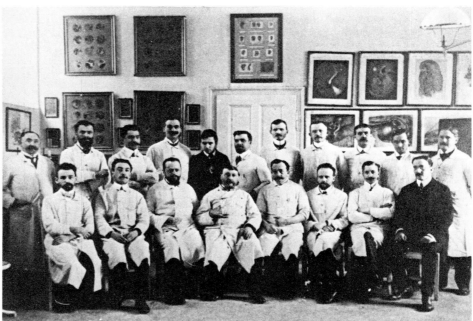

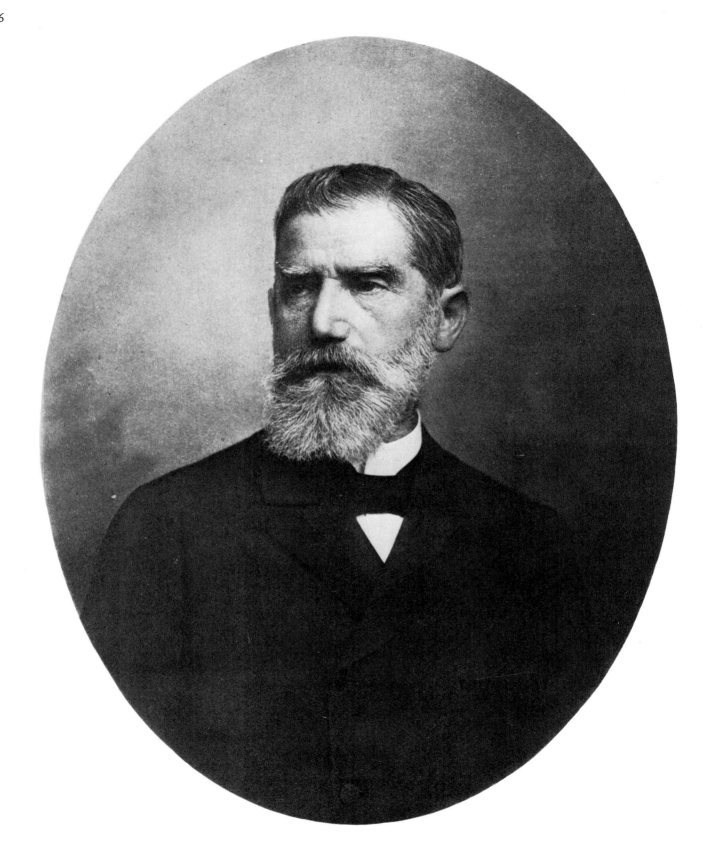

Josef Gruber. Bildnis in mittleren Jahren nach einer undatierten Photographie von Fr. Luckhardt, Wien.

Josef Gruber. Undated photograph of Gruber in middle age; Fr. Luckhardt, Vienna.

Diese Ohrenklinik bestand aus ursprünglich einem Krankenzimmer, das man durch Aufführen einer Zwischenwand in zwei Räume unterteilte. Josef GRUBER (1827–1900) führte die Männerabteilung mit elf, Adam POLITZER die Frauenabteilung mit acht Betten. In diesem kleinen Saal wurde operiert, verbunden und die Untersuchung und Behandlung der immer zahlreicher zuströmenden ambulanten Patienten vorgenommen. Erst im Jahre 1898 kamen zwei neue Räume, ein Ambulanz- und ein Operationsraum, hinzu. „Nie ist eine Klinik mit so wenig Mitteln errichtet worden, nie aus einem einzigen Raum, der POLITZERschen Abteilung ... eine solche mondiale Wirkung ausgegangen. Mit Recht konnte der Minister 1894, als er GRUBER und POLITZER zu Titular-Ordinarien vorschlug, darauf hinweisen, daß ‚fast alle an der Wiener Universität habilitierten Docenten der Ohrenheilkunde, sowie auch der größte Theil der an den Universitäten Deutschlands und anderer Länder als Lehrer der Ohrenheilkunde wirkenden Professoren als Schüler dieser beiden Professoren ... bezeichnet werden'."[24]

Als POLITZER 1907 aus dem Lehramt schied, überreichten ihm seine Schüler eine Abschiedsadresse, die die Namen von 366 Otologen aus Europa, Amerika, Asien, Afrika und Australien enthält. Im Text dazu heißt es: „Nahezu ein halbes Jahrhundert ist vergangen, seitdem Sie als akademischer Lehrer Ihre Vorlesungen über Ohrenheilkunde begonnen haben; ... Nach Tausenden zählen, die von Ihnen an dieser Stelle Unterweisung und Belehrung empfangen – aber unzählbar sind die, die Ihrer Lehre Heilung, Erhaltung der Gesundheit und des Lebens verdanken! ... Aus einem kleinen und wenig geschätzten, etwas abseits gelegenen Spezialgebiete ist in diesen fünfundvierzig Jahren die Ohrenheilkunde ein anerkanntes, ja hervorragendes und umfassendes, vollberechtigtes Fach der Medizin geworden; aus einer Summe einzelner therapeutischer und diagnostischer Kenntnisse ein systematisch geordnetes Gebäude, das, auf gesicherter anatomisch-physiologischer Basis ruhend, die pathologischen Veränderungen und ihre äußeren Zeichen begreift und erklärt und eine rationale Therapie begründet, die sich mit Erfolg an Aufgaben wagen darf, deren Lösung noch vor wenigen Dezennien für unmöglich gehalten wurde."[25] – Und die American Medical Assocation of Vienna ernannte „Hofrath Prof. Adam POLITZER" einstimmig zu ihrem „first honorary member". Doch was aber lag dazwischen!

Dies läßt sich auch anhand des Berufs- und Lebensweges des zweiten Pioniers der Ohrenheilkunde in Österreich, des aus Kosulup in Böhmen gebürtigen Josef GRUBER (1827–1900) zeigen.

Nach seiner Promotion im Jahr 1855 arbeitete GRUBER zunächst als Sekundararzt an verschiedenen Abteilungen des Allgemeinen Krankenhauses, beschäftigte sich aber seit 1860 insbesondere mit der Ohrenheilkunde, „welche er als Autodidact betrieb"[26]. 1862 wurde er zum „Ohrenarzt des k. k. Allgemeinen Krankenhauses" ernannt und erhielt von der Krankenhausdirektion einen kleinen Raum im 1. Hof, in der „historischen Ecke der Ohrenheilkunde",[27] als otiatrisches Ambulatorium zugewiesen; es war dies die erste Fachambulanz in Wien! 1867 erschienen GRUBERS „Anatomisch-physiologische Studien über das Trommelfell und die Gehörknöchelchen", eine rein morphologische Arbeit, auf die sich HELMHOLTZ bezog, als er an seiner „Mechanik der Gehörknöchelchen" arbeitete. In dasselbe Jahr fällt auch die Gründung der ‚Monatsschrift für Ohrenheilkunde' durch GRUBER,

physiological principles, which comprehends and explains pathological changes and their outward signs and offers a rational therapy for them which has successfully dared to attack medical problems whose solution would have been unthinkable only decades ago."[25] The American Medical Association of Vienna unanimously named "Hofrath Prof. Adam POLITZER" their first honorary member. But how far he had come!

This can be shown by taking a look at the career and life of Austria's second pioneer of otology, Josef GRUBER, born in Kosulup in Bohemia.

After having finished his medical studies in 1855, GRUBER worked as *Secundarius* (secondary physician) in various departments of the General Hospital. From 1860 on he was particularly interested in otology, in which he was "self-taught"[26]. In 1862 he was appointed as "Aural Surgeon of the Imperial Royal General Hospital" and was consequently allotted a small room in the first courtyard, in the "historical corner of otology"[27], which was to serve as the first out-patient clinic of otiatry, indeed Vienna's first out-patient clinic of any special field. In 1867 GRUBER's "Anatomical-Physiological Studies of the Tympanic Membrane and the Auditory Ossicles" was published, a purely morphological work to which HELMHOLTZ referred in his study "Mechanics of the Auditory Ossicles". The same year the "Monatsschrift für Ohrenheilkunde" had been jointly founded by GRUBER, Friedrich Eduard Rudolph VOLTOLINI (1819–1889), Friedrich Eugen WEBER-LIEL (1832–1891), and Nicolaus RÜDINGER (1832–1896). In the introduction to the first volume of the "Monatsschrift" WEBER-LIEL expressed the hope that through this journal interest in the "long neglected Cinderella of medicine" would be aroused,[28] for up to that time otiatry had been considered a sterile and hopeless discipline.

In 1871 GRUBER and POLITZER were simultaneously appointed as "titular" associate professors and made joint directors in 1873 of the newly founded University Clinic of Otology. On the occasion of the department's twenty-fifth anniversary in 1899, POLITZER stated retrospectively, and somewhat mellowed: "This measure proved to be constricting for the free development of instruction and totally insufficient for operations, ... Nevertheless, this division, which was unique in the history of medical departments, resulted in advantages which should not be underestimated. It was the trigger for a peaceful rivalry which was extraordinarily fruitful for science."[29] This rivalry was anything but peaceful at the time: in his "Textbook of the Diseases of the Ear" (1870, 2nd edition 1888) which also appeared in English, GRUBER referred to the "so-called" procedure of POLITZER; GRUBER claims to have originated the technique himself in 1862.[30] POLITZER retorted with a caustic reply in his "Textbook of Otology" (1878);[31] that means that the quarrel had lost nothing of its intensity even after the two had been joint directors of Department of Otology for five years. With the introduction of POLITZER's method of tubal inflation of the middle ear with the POLITZER bag, the previous method of catheterization of the tube had become outmoded. His article "On a New Procedure to Cure Deafness Caused by Immobility of the Eustachian Tube" appeared in 1863 in the "Vienna Medical Weekly". For the first time POLITZER reported on the method which he had developed as a natural consequence of the findings he had made in his studies of the anatomy and physiology of the tube: "The method ... is based upon the

gemeinsam mit Friedrich Eduard Rudolph VOLTOLINI (1819–1889), Friedrich Eugen WEBER-LIEL (1832–1891) und Nicolaus RÜDINGER (1832–1896). In seiner Einleitung zum 1. Heft der ‚Monatsschrift' drückte WEBER-LIEL die Hoffnung aus, daß durch diese Zeitschrift das Interesse für das „lang vernachlässigte Aschenbrödel der Medizin"[28] gesteigert werde. Denn bis dahin wurde die Otiatrie als eine sterile und hoffnungslose Disziplin angesehen.

1871 wurden GRUBER und POLITZER gleichzeitig zu unbesoldeten Extraordinarien ernannt und 1873 wurde ihnen gemeinsam die Leitung der neu gegründeten Universitäts-Ohrenklinik übergeben. Wenn POLITZER 1899 aus Anlaß des 25jährigen Bestehens der Ohrenklinik rückblickend feststellt: „Diese Massregel hat sich jedoch als beengend für die freie Entfaltung des Unterrichtes und vollkommen unzureichend für die operative Thätigkeit erwiesen... Demungeachtet hat diese, in der Geschichte der Kliniken einzig dastehende Zweitheilung manche nicht zu unterschätzende Vortheile zur Folge. Sie war der Anlass eines friedlichen Wettstreites, aus dem der Wissenschaft bleibende Errungenschaften erwachsen sind",[29] so war dieser Wettstreit – wie sich belegen läßt – als er ausgetragen wurde, gewiß nicht friedlich: In seinem „Lehrbuch der Ohrenheilkunde" aus dem Jahr 1870 (2. Auflage 1888), das auch in englischer Sprache erschien, spricht GRUBER vom „sogenannten" POLITZERschen Verfahren; GRUBER erhebt dort den Anspruch, das Verfahren 1862 selbst angegeben zu haben.[30] POLITZER entgegnet GRUBER in seinem „Lehrbuch der Ohrenheilkunde", das 1878 in 1. Auflage erschien, in einer Replik,[31] die an Schärfe nichts zu wünschen übrig läßt, d. h., daß der Streit noch aktuell war, als POLITZER und GRUBER schon durch fünf Jahre gemeinsam die Leitung der Ohrenklinik inne hatten! Bekanntlich wurde durch POLITZERS Methode der Lufteinblasung in das Mittelohr mit einem Gummiballon, dem POLITZER-Ballon, dessen Vorgänger, der bis dahin allgemein geübte Katheterismus der Tube, stark zurückgedrängt. Seine diesbezügliche Publikation „Über ein neues Heilverfahren gegen Schwerhörigkeit in Folge von Unwegsamkeit der Eustachischen Ohrtrompete" erschien im Jahr 1863 in der „Wiener Medizinischen Wochenschrift". Zum ersten Mal berichtete POLITZER dort über die Methode, die er in konsequenter Weiterverfolgung der Ideen, die ihm bei seinen Studien über die Anatomie und Physiologie der Tube gekommen waren, ersonnen hatte. Erna LESKY spricht in diesem Zusammenhang von der „schönsten Frucht, die der Ohrenheilkunde aus ihrer neuen Verbindung mit der experimentellen Physiologie erwuchs".[32] POLITZERS Verfahren trat bald seinen Siegeslauf über die Welt an, und TRÖLTSCH behielt recht, als er 1864 darüber urteilte: „Die große Masse der Ungeübten – Ärzte wie Laien – besitzen von nun an die Möglichkeit, eine beträchtliche Reihe von krankhaften Zuständen des Ohres zu beseitigen oder doch zu mildern. Die humane Seite dieses Fortschrittes ist es somit, welche insbesondere nicht hoch genug angeschlagen werden kann und von welcher gerade der Wissenschaft so unendlich viel Förderung entspringen wird."[33] – Weder GRUBER noch August LUCAE (1835–1911) in Berlin konnten durch ihr Unternehmen, den Schluckakt beim Verfahren durch Phonationsakte zu ersetzen und diese Modifikationen als „neue Methoden" zu propagieren,[34] den Ruhm des Erfinders POLITZER schmälern. Eines aber ist klar: so wie der weltbekannt gewordene Prioritätsstreit zwischen den Laryngologen TÜRCK und CZERMAK sich für das Fach selbst positiv auswirkte, so sind auch aus dem fact that condensed air can be blown through the Eustachian tube into the middle ear during an act of swallowing, the naso-pharynx being closed on all sides. The essential novelty of this method, by which it is distinguished from catheterism of the Eustachian tube, lies in the fact that the nozzle of the instrument to be used for condensation of air is introduced only into the anterior portion of the nasal cavity, and thereby introduction of the catheter into the Eustachian tube, which is sometimes impracticable and often disagreeable, is avoided. The closure of the naso-pharynx in this method is effected, behind by the soft palate being closely applied to the posterior pharyngeal wall, and in front by compression of the alae of the nose. At the same time the resistance in the tube is lessened by the act of swallowing, by which the influx of the condensed air into the tympanic cavity is materially facilitated. (This method was suggested by a number of experiments made in reference to the fluctuations in the pressure of air in the tympanic cavity...) The most serviceable instrument for my method is a pyriform balloon, about the size of the doubled fist, which is furnished with a slightly curved tabular nozzle. To avoid bleeding, which is frequently produced by the immediate impact of the stiff nozzle upon the pituitary membrane, the connection between the balloon and the nozzle is effected by the insertion of a short elastic india-rubber tube. The details of the method are the following: The patient, seated in a chair, takes a little water into his mouth, which he is required to swallow when told. (The use of water is by no means absolutely necessary in all cases during the application of my method, which I often perform during a simple act of swallowing, the effect of an energetic act of deglutition being the same as that of drinking water. Sometimes, however, the simple act of swallowing is less powerful, and not only is deglutition in such cases materially facilitated by drinking water, but the lumen of the Eustachian tube is also more widened by the powerful contraction of the naso-pharyngeal muscles, and the effect of the injected air is increased. MIOT gives the patient a small piece of sugar instead of water, by which salivation is produced, facilitating the act of swallowing.) The surgeon, standing on the patient's right, introduces the nozzle of the Politzer-bag one cm. into the corresponding orifice, and then compresses with the left thumb and forefinger the alae of the nose closely around the instrument. The patient is next told to perform an act of swallowing, and at the same moment the surgeon expels the air from the inflating-bag with his right hand. By the condensation of air, produced in the naso-pharynx in this manner, the closure effected by the soft palate is forced open, and its vibrations give rise to a dull gurgling noise which frequently, if not always, may be taken as an indication that the air has entered into the middle ear. The majority of patients experience at the same time the subjective sensation of a stream of air entering both tympanic cavities. If this sensation of air streaming into the tympanic cavity is more pronounced on one side, it is in many cases due to the difference in the permeability of the tubes; but if this sensation be quite absent it must by no means be concluded that the air has not reached the middle ear, as not infrequently the sensibility of the mucous membrane of the tympanic cavity in aural patients has become so diminished that even during catheterism the current of air in the middle ear is not felt." As regards the therapeutic value of his method, POLITZER states: "My method of inflating the tympanic cavity is rarely less effective

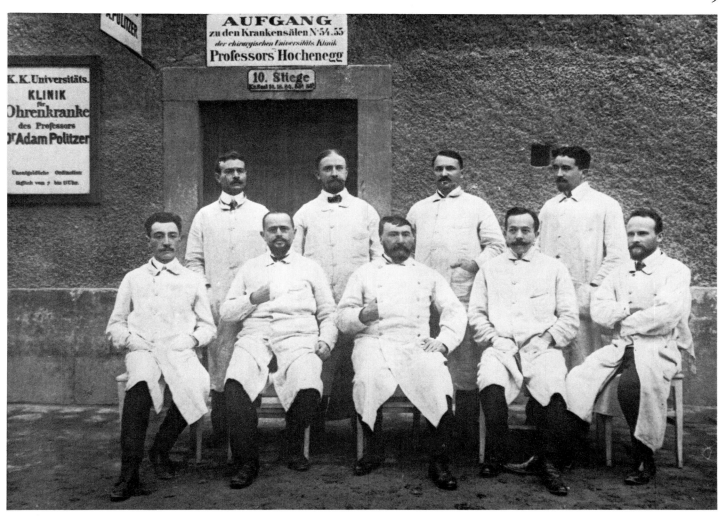

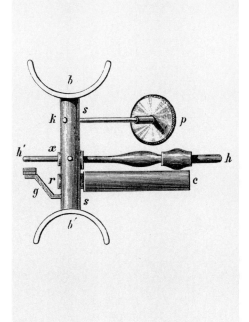

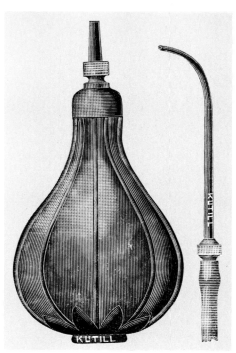

Oben: Politzer mit Assistenten vor der Ohrenklinik.
Links unten: Der „einheitliche Hörmesser" von A. Politzer zur Präzisierung der Hörschärfe.
Rechts unten: Ballon zur Luftdusche mit Tubenkatheter (Politzer-Ballon).

Top: Politzer and assistants in front of the Clinic of Otology.
Bottom left: Politzer's universal acoumeter for testing the acuteness of hearing. It consisted of a horizontal steel cylinder (c), 28 mm. long and 4.5 mm. thick, connected with a perpendicular vulcanite column (s) by means of a tight screw. Above the place of attachment of the steel cylinder the percussion hammer (h, h') is attached. This is movable on its long axis, and produces the tone by falling upon the steel cylinder.
Bottom right: Politzer's air-bag for making the Eustachian tube permeable. Politzer's original hand air-bag (1863) consisted chiefly of an ordinary air-bag, such as had been used for forcing air through the Eustachian catheter. Instead of the conical tip of the ordinary hand air-bag, the instrument devised by Politzer was supplied with a somewhat bulbous tip, to which was attached a piece of black rubber tube 8 cm. long, which formed a pliable connection between the air-bag and the nose piece.

Wettstreit zwischen POLITZER und GRUBER „der Wissenschaft manche Errungenschaften erwachsen". War auch die „Zweitheilung in der Geschichte der Kliniken einzig" – es wurde der zweigeteilten Klinik auch nur eine Assistentenstelle genehmigt[35] – so hätte man andernfalls – wie dies 1875 aufgrund einer besonderen Situation in der Psychiatrie geschah – zwei Kliniken für ein Fach schaffen müssen, das damals weder obligatorisch noch ein Prüfungsfach war. So aber trennte man jenen ebenerdig im I. Hof des Allgemeinen Krankenhauses gelegenen Raum, in dem GRUBER seit 1862 allein sein otiatrisches Ambulatorium hatte, durch eine „Scheidewand in zwei Räume", d. h. GRUBER war der eigentlich Leidtragende bei der Errichtung der Klinik. Trocken heißt es dazu im Statthalterei-Erlaß: „Bei dem Umstande als sich die beiden Ohrenärzte und a. o. Professoren Dr. GRUBER und Dr. POLLITZER [sic] um die fortschrittliche Entwicklung der Ohrenheilkunde an der Wiener Universität in ebenbürtiger Weise verdient gemacht haben, fand der Herr Minister gleichzeitig anzuordnen, daß die Leitung dieser Klinik unter die beiden vorgenannten Professoren in der Art getheilt werde, daß Professor Dr. GRUBER die Abtheilung für ohrenkranke Männer, Professor Dr. POLITZER dagegen die Abtheilung für ohrenkranke Frauen übernimmt."[36] – Beim Ausscheiden GRUBERS im Jahr 1898 aus der Klinik wegen Erreichung der Altersgrenze – 1894 waren er und POLITZER zu unbesoldeten Ordinarien ernannt worden – wurde GRUBER von der Unterrichtsverwaltung für seine „erfolgreiche, ohne irgendeine Vergütung durch 35 Jahre fortgesetzte lehramtliche Thätigkeit" die allerhöchste Anerkennung ausgesprochen.[37]
Es spricht für POLITZER, daß er beim Ausscheiden aus dem Lehramt in seiner Rede GRUBER als einen Kollegen würdigte, „dem ein hervorragender Anteil an den an der Ohrenklinik erzielten Erfolgen gebührt. Seine anerkannten Leistungen auf dem Gebiete der Ohrenanatomie und der praktischen Ohrenheilkunde, sein hervorragendes Lehrtalent und sein humanes Wirken als Arzt, sein unermüdlicher Eifer für die Förderung unseres Spezialfaches wird den Namen GRUBERS für alle Zeiten mit der Geschichte der Ohrenklinik eng verknüpfen."[38] Die Worte POLITZERS, die er in dieser Rede an die Assistenten richtete, daß „neben Talent und Begabung Fleiß und Ausdauer die unumgänglichen Postulate erfolgreichen Schaffens sind", gelten ohne Einschränkung auch für GRUBER: sein Arbeitsverzeichnis nennt mehr als 150 Titel und im Jahr 1876 verzeichnet sein Ambulanzprotokoll die Nummer 91.000! Sie bergen auch den Schlüssel zu POLITZERS eigenem Erfolg: Die Ernennung zum Armen-Ohrenarzt der Stadt Wien (1863) öffnete ihm die Tore zu den Versorgungshäusern und gab ihm die Möglichkeit, „durch 30 Jahre ... eine große Reihe von Krankheitsformen des Gehörorgans, die man in den Spitälern nur äußerst selten findet, zu beobachten und durch die Autopsie post mortem zu verifizieren. Ich brauche nur auf die reiche Ausbeute langjährig beobachteter Adhäsivprozesse im Mittelohre, auf die große Serie der Ohrcholesteatome und auf die Otosklerose hinzuweisen, durch welch letztere erst die anatomische Grundlage einer in der Praxis so häufig vorkommenden Ohraffektion erkannt wurde."[39] Dieses große Krankenmaterial und natürlich auch das des Allgemeinen Krankenhauses bildete die Grundlage für sein 1865 erschienenes Werk „Die Beleuchtungsbilder des Trommelfelles im gesunden und kranken Zustande". Dabei kamen ihm „Talent und Begabung", über beides verfügte er in großem

than the air-douche with the catheter, and is frequently even more so, possessing considerable advantages over catheterism. They are: 1. The simplicity of its application, which enables the practitioner who is not familiar with catheterism to effect, in many cases, the permeability of the Eustachian tube, and to treat with success a number of affections of the middle ear. 2. The possibility of injecting air into the middle ear in the treatment of many cases in which catheterism of the Eustachian tube is very difficult or impossible. The application of my method of inflation is specially serviceable in the case of children who suffer very frequently from great dullness of hearing in the course of acute or chronic nasopharyngeal catarrhs, with hypertrophy of the tonsils, owing to consecutive swelling of mucous membrane of the Eustachian tube and effusion in the tympanic cavity. The method can also be applied in the congenital or acquired deformities and diseases of the naso-pharynx which prevent the introduction of the catheter. But even when the nasal cavity is normal, this method will be exclusively employed for effecting the permeability of the Eustachian tube in persons who object to the introduction of the catheter, in nervous individuals, in aged people, and in convalescents from severe illness, in whose cases the permeability of the Eustachian tube requires to be established on account of accumulation of secretion in the middle ear, but whose weakness and irritability do not allow of the use of the catheter. 3. The application of my method in all those cases in which catheterism of the Eustachian tube can be dispensed with. If it is, therefore, necessary to effect the permeability of the tube by a current of air, this method is always to be preferred to catheterism, because thus the unpleasant sensation caused by the latter proceeding is avoided, because the local irritation of the mucous membrane of the tube by immediate contact with the catheter does not take place; and lastly, because the permeability of both Eustachian tubes can be effected simultaneously. But I must repeat here most emphatically, that it frequently happens that catheterism of the tube, as a diagnostic and as a therapeutic agent, cannot be replaced by any other method, especially if the catheter is required as a conducting-tube for the injection of fluids and for the introduction of bougies into the middle ear. 4. My method has also the advantage that on account of its easy application it is well adapted for self-treatment, especially in those chronic affections of the middle ear in which, after the surgical treatment has terminated, inflation of the middle ear is from time to time necessary to retain the improvement effected in the hearing and to prevent a relapse." Erna LESKY speaks in this regard of the "most valuable result of otology's new relation with experimental physiology."[32] POLITZER's method began its triumphal race around the globe and TRÖLTSCH was right in proclaiming in 1864: "The great masses of the unpracticed – physicians as well as laymen – now have the possibility to eliminate or at least to soothe a considerable number of pathological conditions of the ear. It is therefore the humane aspect of this achievement which cannot be praised highly enough, and from which science will receive so much impetus."[33] – Neither GRUBER nor August LUCAE (1835–1911) in Berlin succeeded in lessening POLITZER's fame by propagating modifications of POLITZER's procedure as "their new methods".[34] One thing is clear, however: just as the worldwide priority dispute between the laryngologists TÜRCK and CZERMAK eventually worked to the benefit of the special discipline laryngology, so was the rivalry between

Maße, zugute: POLITZER fertigte selbst die zeichnerischen Grundlagen für dieses Werk, für das Carl HEITZMANN (1836–1896), auf den später noch zurückzukommen sein wird, die Chromlithographien ausführte, an. Als 1896 POLITZERS „Atlas der Beleuchtungsbilder des Trommelfelles im gesunden und kranken Zustande" erschien, waren die zwei Tafeln und 24 Beleuchtungsbilder des Trommelfelles des Jahres 1865 zu 14 Tafeln mit 392 Reproduktionen von Trommelfellbildern angewachsen, obwohl auch sie nur eine Auswahl des riesigen Materials darstellen. Die reichen und gründlichen Erkenntnisse auf pathologisch-anatomischem Gebiet blieben nicht ohne ausschlaggebenden und bestimmenden Einfluß auf die Diagnostik und Therapie der Ohrenerkrankungen. Das gründliche Studium der Trommelfellveränderungen, das mit Einführung des Stirnreflektors wesentlich erleichtert wurde, und über das POLITZERS Atlas besonderes Zeugnis ablegt, ermöglichte eine richtige Verwertung des otoskopischen Bildes für Erkennung, Deutung und Beurteilung der Mittelohrerkrankungen. Wenn der Otologe imstande ist, aus den jeweiligen Trommelfellveränderungen sichere Schlüsse auf das pathologische Geschehen im Mittelohr, in der Eustachischen Röhre und im Warzenfortsatz zu ziehen, so ist dies der gründlichen, auf jedes noch so gering scheinende Detail hinweisenden Untersuchung POLITZERS zu danken.
Es gibt, so Gustav ALEXANDER (1873–1932), kein Gebiet der Otologie, auf dem POLITZER nicht Grundlegendes geschaffen hätte.⁴⁰ Insgesamt veröffentlichte er weit über einhundert wissenschaftliche Arbeiten, die sich u. a. mit der Diagnose und Therapie des sekretorischen Katarrhs, mit der pathologischen Anatomie bei Taubstummen, mit Veränderungen bei Labyrintheiterungen, bei Panotitis, Leukämie, Lues und Typhus beschäftigen. Zur Feststellung der Tubendurchlässigkeit gab POLITZER einen Stimmgabeltest an: Der Ton einer vor die Nase gehaltenen Stimmgabel wird als schwacher, gleichmäßiger Ton gehört. Wenn der Patient schluckt, wird der Ton während des Schluckens bei durchgängiger Tube deutlich lauter.
1878 erschien POLITZERS „Lehrbuch der Ohrenheilkunde", ein Werk, in dem in klassischer Form die wissenschaftliche wie die praktische Seite der Otologie seiner Zeit niedergelegt ist, und das zu einem Standardwerk des Faches durch Jahrzehnte hindurch wurde; es erlebte bis zum Jahre 1908 fünf Auflagen und wurde ins Französische, Englische und Spanische übersetzt.
In seinem Vorwort zur 1981 erschienenen Übersetzung des ersten Bandes von POLITZERS zweibändiger „Geschichte der Ohrenheilkunde" ins Englische meint E. H. MAJER treffend: „Für jeden Otologen ist die Kenntnis der Entwicklung der Fachgeschichte bis in die Neuzeit sehr lehrreich. Wenn sich auch unsere heutige Grundlagenforschung kompliziertester technischer Apparate und genauester biochemischer Untersuchungsmethoden bedienen kann, so ist es doch von besonderem Interesse, in POLITZERS Werk Näheres über die Ansichten der alten Völker, der Griechen und Römer, über Ohrerkrankungen zu hören und die zunehmenden Kenntnisse der Anatomie und Physiologie des Gehörorganes bis in die Neuzeit zu verfolgen. ... Es ist äußerst reizvoll, die Entwicklung der Diagnostik- und Therapiemöglichkeiten mit den primitivsten Hilfsmitteln bis in die Zeit POLITZERS zu betrachten. ... Wer POLITZERS Geschichte der Ohrenheilkunde studiert, denkt unwillkürlich an Richard WAGNERS Meistersinger: ‚Vergeßt die alten Meister nicht und ehret ihre Kunst.'"⁴¹ –

POLITZER and GRUBER extraordinarily fruitful for otology. There is no doubt that the division of GRUBER's one-room otological out-patient department into two rooms by erecting a "partition-wall" was "unique in the history of medicine", as POLITZER stated, with only one assistant for the two heads.³⁵ On the other hand, the establishment of two departments of otology would have meant having two departments for a speciality which was neither compulsory nor an examination subject. In 1875 such treatment was accorded only to psychiatry in Vienna, and only because of a very special situation. In this new arrangement GRUBER was the one who suffered most. He had been the exclusive head of his department since 1862, but now he had to share this room with POLITZER. In the Ministry of Education's decree this arrangement dryly reads: "In view of the fact that the professors Dr. GRUBER and Dr. POLLITZER [sic] have both been equally successful in the development of otology at the University of Vienna it is decreed that both be entrusted with the direction of the clinic in such a way that professor Dr. GRUBER shall head the department for male ear patients while professor Dr. POLLITZER shall head the department for female ear patients."³⁶ – When GRUBER left the department in 1898 on reaching retirement age (in 1894 he and POLITZER had been appointed unpaid full professors), he received the most sincere acknowledgement from the Ministry of Education for his "successful work as a teacher for 35 years without any compensation."³⁷ It speaks for POLITZER that in his valedictory lecture he honored GRUBER by giving him credit as a colleague "to whom a large part of the success of the Clinic of Otology is due. His acknowledged achievements concerning the anatomy of the ear and practical otology, his outstanding talents as a teacher and his humane work as a physician, his tireless devotion to the promotion of our specialty will forever tie GRUBER's name to the history of the Clinic of Otology."³⁸ POLITZER's words in the same lecture, addressed to his assistants, that "apart from talents and natural gifts, industry and perseverance are the most absolute prerequisites for successful work," are also true for GRUBER: the four pages of small print which list more than 150 publications demonstrate an astonishing number of works, and by 1876 his out-patients numbered 91,000! These words are also the key to POLITZER's own success: as otologist to the municipality of Vienna – he had been appointed "Town Physician to the Poor" in 1863 – he was given access to a vast amount of clinical and post-mortem material in Vienna's nursing homes. "For thirty years I was able to observe patients there, follow up my findings, and subsequently check them in post-mortem examinations. I need only point out the large number of adhesive processes in the middle ear which I was able to observe, or the great number of cholesteatomas of the ear and cases of otosclerosis due to the latter of which it was possible to discover the anatomical basis of a very common affection of the ear."³⁹ POLITZER made excellent use of this extensive material in preparing his book "Pictures of the Tympanic Membrane in Health and Disease" (Vienna, 1865), and since he was also a master of the pen and brush, POLITZER himself made the sketches for this work, for which Carl HEITZMANN (1836–1896) drew the chromolithographs. When this work was rewritten in 1896 as "Atlas of the Tympanic Membrane in Health and Disease", clinical categories, i.e., different types of acute and chronic inflammation of the tympanic membrane, determined the classification. The 1865 edition with

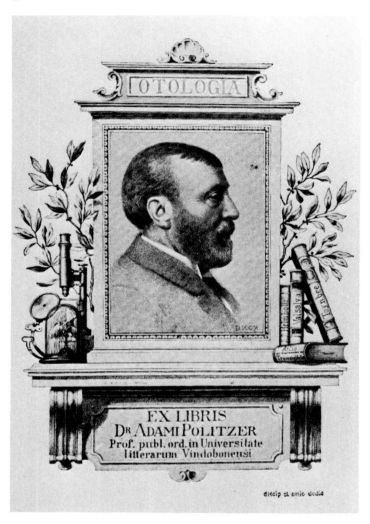

Exlibris Adam Politzers.

Exlibris of Adam Politzer.

Das Interesse in den Vereinigten Staaten von Amerika an POLITZER bis in die jüngste Gegenwart kommt nicht von ungefähr. In seinem Nachruf auf POLITZER erklärte STUEVER aus New York im Namen der Ärzte Amerikas unter anderem: „Wenn in irgendein Land die Schule POLITZERS eingedrungen ist, wenn sie irgendwo mit Vorliebe aufgenommen wurde, so ist dies in Amerika der Fall; denn die amerikanische Schule ist eins mit der Wiener Schule."[42]

POLITZERS Lieblingsgebiet war stets die Anatomie und pathologische Anatomie des Ohres. Unter dem Einfluß von Joseph HYRTL (1810–1894), einem „der glänzendsten Repräsentanten der vergleichenden Anatomie des Gehörganges", wie POLITZER ihn selbst in seiner „Geschichte der Ohrenheilkunde" (Band 1, Seite 388) apostrophiert, ROKITANSKYS und TOYNBEES beschäftigte er sich vor allem mit der normalen und pathologischen Anatomie des Schläfenbeines und war auch ein Meister der Präpariertechnik. POLITZERS Präparate waren bald international so gefragt wie diejenigen HYRTLS und sechzig seiner künstlerisch ausgeführten Präparate wurden 1876 an das Mütter Museum in Philadelphia geliefert. Als in Wien bekannt wurde, daß diese Sammlung an das Mütter Museum verkauft worden war, erschienen Karikaturen in Wiener Tageszeitungen, die POLITZER als gemeinen Dieb von Schläfenbeinen darstellten. Um die Öffentlichkeit zu beruhigen,

two tables and 24 pictures was expanded to 14 tables with 392 chromolithographic reproductions of findings in the tympanic membrane. However, even these were only a selection of the enormous amount of material which showed POLITZER to be a complete clinician who made contemporary morphological as well as experimental methods subservient to the goals of otology, which in the meantime had matured into a specialty in its own right. Due to POLITZER's painstaking works, paying attention even to the smallest detail, the otologist now is able to diagnose the pathological processes in the middle ear, in the Eustachian tube, and in the mastoid process from changes in the eardrum.

According to Gustav ALEXANDER (1873–1932) there is no branch of otology to which POLITZER did not contribute considerably.[40] He published scientific papers (103 in all) dealing with almost all fields of otology, including studies on the diagnosis and therapy of serous otitis media, the pathological anatomy in deaf-mutism, alterations caused by labyrinth suppuration, panotitis, leukemia, syphilis, and typhoid fever. For determining tubal patency POLITZER developed a tuning-fork test: the tone of a tuning-fork held in front of the nose of a patient is recognized as a weak and even tone. When swallowing the sound is heard louder if the tube is permeable. In 1878 POLITZER's "Textbook of Otology" appeared, which

50 Jahre „Archiv für Ohrenheilkunde" und dessen Gründer: A. v. Tröltsch (Würzburg), A. Politzer (Wien) und H. Schwartze (Halle).
Aus: Archiv für Ohrenheilkunde, Band 96 (1914).

50 Years "Archives of Otology" (1864–1914) and its founders: A. v. Tröltsch (Würzburg), A. Politzer (Vienna), and H. Schwartze (Halle).
From the "Archives of Otology", vol. 96 (1914).

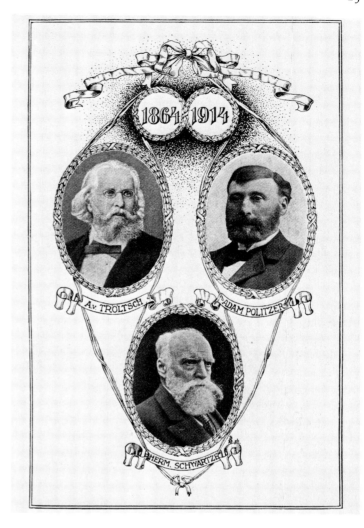

verlangte POLITZER eine Bestätigung des College of Physicians in Philadelphia, die klarstellte, daß er nur für die Herstellung der Präparate und für seinen Arbeitsaufwand entschädigt worden war.[43] Die Einführung und weitere Vervollkommnung der Präpariertechnik des Schläfenbeines ermöglichten nicht nur ein ganz genaues Studium der normal anatomischen Details; sie brachten auch wichtige Aufklärungen über die feineren geweblichen Veränderungen bei Erkrankungen des Gehörorgans. Es ist POLITZERS Verdienst, die Bedeutung der Histologie für die Untersuchungen des Schläfenbeines frühzeitig erkannt und sie zur Grundlage des Studiums der pathologischen Anatomie des Gehörorganes gemacht zu haben.

Im Jahr 1893 reiste POLITZER in die Vereinigten Staaten. In seinem Vortrag auf dem Panamerikanischen Kongreß in Washington betonte er, daß die bisher als „trockene Mittelohrkatarrhe" bezeichneten Fälle mit progredienter Schwerhörigkeit nicht durch eine Erkrankung der Mittelohrschleimhaut, sondern durch eine Erkrankung der Labyrinthkapsel bedingt seien; er hat somit als erster das klinische Bild der typischen Otosklerose präzisiert. Im Rahmen dieses Aufenthaltes in den Vereinigten Staaten stattete er auch dem Mütter Museum in Philadelphia einen Besuch ab und zeigte sich zufrieden über den guten Zustand der von ihm stammenden Präparate. Seine

was a standard work for this field for decades. Five editions appeared up to 1908 and they were translated into French, English and Spanish. In his preface to the first volume of POLITZER's "History of Otology", which appeared in an English translation in 1981, E. H. MAJER states: "Despite the profound changes in otology brought about by the introduction of antibiotics and microsurgery, it is still vital for each otologist to be acquainted with the evolution of our specialty. An Austrian proverb states: 'He who studies history becomes wise.' It is wisdom, above all, that is needed today. We otologists stand posed on the threshold of major advances; microelectronics and biochemical research hold great promise. We must, however, realize that great forward strides are made possible only through the labors of countless generations of physicians of the past. Technological innovation is usually at the end of a chain of scholarly endeavors lasting decades or even centuries. A line from 'Die Meistersinger' comes to mind: 'Remember and venerate the old masters and their art.'"[41] – It does not come as a surprise that there is still a vivid interest in POLITZER and his work in the United States of America, for STUEVER (New York) stated in his commemorative address that any country which, like America, formally accepted the POLITZER school became identical with the Vienna school in its principles.[42]

Technik des Präparierens läßt sich im Detail nachlesen in seinem Werk „Die anatomische und histologische Zergliederung des menschlichen Gehörorgans im normalen und kranken Zustande für Anatomen, Ohrenärzte und Studierende" aus dem Jahr 1889, das in englischer Übersetzung („The Anatomical and Histological Dissection of the Human Ear in the Normal and Diseased Condition") 1891 erschien. – Noch heute werden POLITZERS und auch HYRTLS Präparate, deren Erhaltungszustand nach wie vor gut ist, im Mütter Museum in Philadelphia den Besuchern gezeigt. Für die Otologen stellt diese Sammlung ein Vermächtnis dar, das nichts von seiner Wirkung verloren hat.

POLITZER war auch ein glänzender Vortragender, wobei ihm seine Sprachbegabung – er beherrschte neben der deutschen und ungarischen auch die englische, französische, italienische und spanische Sprache – zugute kam. Hatten zunächst nur vier Hörer seinen ersten Kurs besucht, so wurden sie während seiner 46jährigen Lehrtätigkeit außer von den inskribierten Studenten von über 7.000 ausländischen Hörern frequentiert. Erna LESKY weist darauf hin,[44] daß dieser Lehrerfolg nicht nur in der außergewöhnlichen Begabung POLITZERS als Lehrer zu suchen ist, sondern er ist „das Ergebnis der von unseren Meistern SKODA, OPPOLZER, HEBRA, ARLT u. a. überkommenen Lehrmethode, an der die klinischen Vorstände unserer Facultät noch jetzt festhalten und der die Wiener Schule von jeher ihren Ruf verdankt. Es ist dies der unmittelbar an die Krankenbeobachtung anknüpfende, von jedem überflüssigen, theoretischen Beiwerk losgelöste Unterricht, durch den sich dem Lernenden das für den realen Boden seiner Praxis unentbehrliche Krankheitsbild unauslöschlich dem Gedächtnis einprägt. Diese Methode darf aber keineswegs als eine unorganische Schilderung von Krankheitsfällen angesehen werden, sie ist vielmehr eine auf streng wissenschaftlicher Grundlage sich aufbauende, kritische Analyse der Krankheitserscheinungen und der Krankheitsvorgänge, durch die der Lernende zum selbständigen Denken und, bei günstiger Veranlagung, zum Forschen angeregt wird. Mit Genugthuung können wir constatieren, dass diese Lehrmethode der Wiener Schule auch an mehreren Facultäten des Auslandes Eingang gefunden hat."[45] Hier setzte POLITZER in einer Schule fort, die von Anton DE HAEN (1704–1776) bis Johann OPPOLZER reicht, und von der der Unterricht am Krankenbett in klassischer Weise zu einer Kunst eigener Art ausgebildet worden war. Die eben zitierten Sätze stehen in der Rede POLITZERS, die er am 21. Jänner 1899 anläßlich der Eröffnung der neuen Räume der otiatrischen Klinik – nach GRUBERS Ausscheiden war POLITZER im Jahr 1898 zum alleinigen Vorstand der Klinik ernannt worden – hielt. Die Klinik wurde um einen eigenen Ambulanz- und einen Operationsraum erweitert, und POLITZER hoffte, daß dadurch „künftighin eine freiere Entfaltung des otiatrischen Unterrichtes und der operativen Thätigkeit" gesichert wäre, denn „von jetzt ab soll der otiatrische Unterricht, welcher bisher trotz der ungünstigen räumlichen Verhältnisse den Wettstreit mit den prunkvoll ausgestatteten Ohrenkliniken des Auslandes ehrenvoll bestand, in einer dem hohen Range unserer Universität würdigen Weise gepflegt und die Krankenzimmer der Ohrenklinik, unberührt von dem lärmenden Getriebe der ambulatorischen Kranken, ihrer eigentlichen Bestimmung zugeführt werden".[46] Zu der Zeit betrug übrigens die Zahl der jährlich ambulant Behandelten 15.000, die Zahl der Mastoid- und Radikaloperationen durchschnittlich 400 pro Jahr.[47]

Influenced by HYRTL and ROKITANSKY in Vienna, and TOYNBEE in London, POLITZER especially occupied himself with the normal and pathological anatomy of the temporal bone. He was also a master of the dissection technique. Sixty of his beautifully prepared temporal bones were delivered to the Mütter Museum in Philadelphia in 1876. When the news reached Vienna that the collection had been sold to a museum in America, POLITZER was depicted in cartoons appearing in local papers as a common thief snatching temporal bones for sale. To appease the public, POLITZER requested a letter from The College of Physicians of Philadelphia stating that this payment was for the mounting and preparing of specimens rather than obtaining them.[43] The collection of temporal bone dissections is still housed today at the Mütter Museum in a wooden case with each bone mounted on a small pedestal covered by a bell jar. The methods of securing the bones and producing the dissections have been described in detail by POLITZER in "Die anatomische und histologische Zergliederung des menschlichen Gehörorgans im normalen und kranken Zustande für Anatomen, Ohrenärzte und Studierende", published in 1889, with the English version, "The Anatomical and Histological Dissection of the Human Ear in the Normal and Diseased Condition", appearing in 1891. In the introduction POLITZER writes: "The first recorded attempt to arrive at a knowledge of the organ of hearing by the assistance of dissection, dates back to the sixteenth and seventeenth centuries, when the revival of the science of anatomy gave so great an impetus to the study of such phases of medical science. In spite of this, however, FALLOPIUS, Ph. INGRASSIAS, Bartholomeo EUSTACHIO, VALSALVA, CASSEBOHM, CASSERIUS, FABRICIUS AB AQUAPENDENTE, have transmitted to posterity but few practical hints relative to the dissection of the human ear. From this period, down to a comparatively recent date, the subject has hardly attracted that attention and consideration which its importance merits. TOYNBEE, HYRTL, Van den BROEK, SAPPEY, Von TRÖLTSCH, KÖLLIKER, VOLTOLINI, MOOS, ZAUFAL, BRUNNER, RÜDINGER, ZUCKERKANDL, LUCAE, WENDT, SCHALLE, SCHWALBE and others, while they have given to the world an elaborate wealth of detail relative to aural anatomy, have hardly treated the matter with that comprehensive scope which is so necessary to enable students to obtain a grasp of the whole subject. This fact, combined with the expressed wish of many of those who attended my lectures, has induced me to venture to bring together in a clear manner the result of modern scientific research in this most interesting field of anatomical inquiry. For the past twenty-five years I have pursued, during the intervals of leisure from my professional otological work, an uninterrupted study of the normal and pathological anatomy and histology of the ear, and I may say that the resultant knowledge and experience thus gained, together with matter collected for lectures, form a basis which has proved invaluable to me in preparing the present work. In dealing with the various methods of preparation which are employed in the anatomical and histological dissection of the ear, I have endeavoured to be as minute as possible, and the aim kept in view has been the finding and the representing with facility the various parts of the organ in their respective positions. The same section of the work treats of the best methods of preserving a collection of preparations, whether wet or dry, and the means to be employed in adjusting and mounting them. I have contented myself, relative to making the technical proceeding available for patholo-

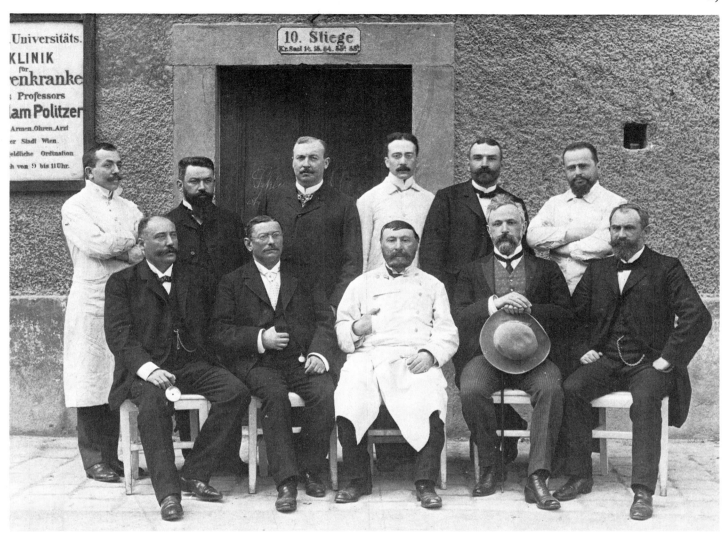

Oben: Adam Politzer mit befreundeten Ohrenärzten.
1. Reihe v. links: Koebel, Bloch, Politzer, Vohsen, Rudloff.
2. Reihe v. links: Neumann, Manasse, Röpke, Frey, Hinsberg, Alexander.
Photographie, Wien 1903.
Unten: Adam Politzer (2. Reihe, Mitte) auf dem Kongreß „Eye, Ear, Nose and Throat". Photographie, Wien 1905.

Top: Adam Politzer and colleagues.
First row, from left to right: Koebel, Bloch, Politzer, Vohsen, Rudloff.
Second row, from left to right: Neumann, Manasse, Röpke, Frey, Hinsberg, Alexander. Photograph, Vienna, 1903.
Bottom: Adam Politzer (in the middle of the second row) and participants of the congress "Eye, Ear, Nose and Throat". Photograph, Vienna, 1905.

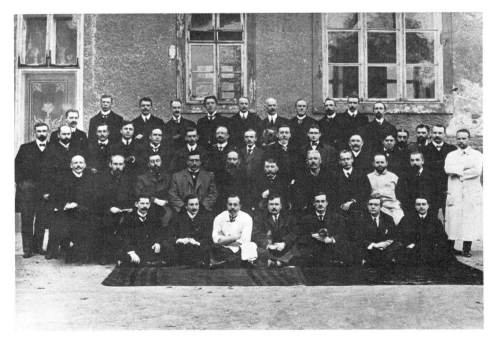

Im Jahr 1907 mußte POLITZER mit Erreichung der Altersgrenze von seiner Klinik Abschied nehmen. Ein Jahr vorher hatte er beim Deutschen Otologenkongreß in seinem Vortrag über den Stand der Ohrenheilkunde erklärt: „Wir dürfen nur auf jene chirurgischen Eingriffe hinweisen, welche sich den höchsten Aufgaben der modernen Chirurgie anreihen lassen: Ich meine die operative Behandlung der otitischen Hirnabszesse und der thrombosierten Hirnblutleiter: Eingriffe, durch die bereits zahlreiche, dem sicheren Tode geweihte Existenzen dem Leben erhalten wurden."[48]

Eine große Zahl von Studenten und Ärzten aus der ganzen Welt hat POLITZER ausgebildet und seine Wiener Klinik war ein Mekka der Ohrenheilkunde. Durch sein wissenschaftliches Werk hat er sich ein unvergängliches Denkmal gesetzt und von allen seinen Zeitgenossen hat er den Ausbau der Ohrenheilkunde am nachhaltigsten gefördert. Von großer Bedeutung für das Fach war auch die Gründung des Archivs für Ohrenheilkunde im Jahr 1864, des ersten deutschsprachigen Fachorgans, durch Anton Friedrich VON TRÖLTSCH (1829–1890), Hermann SCHWARTZE (1837–1910) und POLITZER und 1895 die Gründung der Österreichischen Otologischen Gesellschaft durch ihn gemeinsam mit Josef GRUBER und Viktor VON URBANTSCHITSCH (1847–1921).

Seine Arbeitsweise und Forschungstätigkeit pflanzte sich von ihm auf seine Schüler und Mitarbeiter zu deren Schülern weiter fort, und POLITZER konnte bei seinem Ausscheiden aus dem Lehramt feststellen: „Wenn ich heute die stattliche Reihe meiner Assistenten überblicke, die mir vom Beginn meiner klinischen Tätigkeit hilfreich zur Seite standen, so erfüllt es mich mit Stolz und Freude, daß der Mehrzahl von ihnen, als der Frucht ihres wissenschaftlichen Strebens, die Ehre, als Lehrer zu wirken, zuteil geworden ist."[49] Noch zu seinen Lebzeiten wurden an folgenden Wiener Krankenanstalten eigene Ambulatorien bzw. Abteilungen für Ohrenkrankheiten errichtet und mit ehemaligen Assistenten POLITZERS besetzt: 1892 wurde Benjamin GOMPERZ (1861–1935) Leiter der Ohrenabteilung des Ersten öffentlichen Kinder-Krankeninstitutes; er widmete eine selbständige Untersuchung der "Pathologie und Therapie der Mittelohrentzündungen im Säuglingsalter" (Wien 1906). Daniel KAUFMANN (1864–1919) war von 1898 bis 1908 Vorstand der Ohrenabteilung des Kaiser-Franz-Joseph-Ambulatoriums, wo er 1909 von Hugo FREY (1873–1951) abgelöst wurde. FREY arbeitete über die Physiologie des Schalleitungsapparates und hielt seit 1900 klinische Operationskurse, die insbesondere von amerikanischen Ärzten stark frequentiert wurden. Diese Abteilung übernahm 1912 Heinrich NEUMANN (1873–1939), der 1919 zum Vorstand der Ohrenklinik ernannt wurde. Ferdinand ALT (1867–1923) gründete als Ohrenarzt des Rudolfspitals und des Wiedner Krankenhauses 1900 an beiden Anstalten Ambulatorien mit der Erlaubnis, operative Fälle an den chirurgischen Abteilungen unterzubringen. Er widmete sich vor allem den beruflichen Schädigungen des Gehörorganes.

POLITZER war aber nicht nur der Begründer des Spezialfaches in Wien, er wurde und blieb bis heute mit seiner zweibändigen „Geschichte der Ohrenheilkunde" ihr maßgeblicher Historiker. Seine an den Beginn des Werkes gestellten Sätze: „Die Geschichte der Medizin hat bis vor kurzem nur wenig Beachtung gefunden. Erst in neuerer Zeit hat das gesteigerte historische Interesse ... in weiteren ärztlichen Kreisen Eingang gefunden. Auch hier beginnt die Ueberzeugung durch-

gico-anatomical study, merely with the main features, because the manifold morbid changes in the middle ear, and the frequently complicated alterations in the temporal bone, would render it impossible to give a description of all cases occurring in dissection. I am convinced that the best means of hitting upon the right method of preparation in complicated pathological cases, is to be thoroughly acquainted with the technicalities of the work of dissecting the normal ear."

In 1893 POLITZER visited the United States. In his lecture given at the Pan-American Congress held in Washington, D.C., he explained that the so-called 'dry catarrhal otitis' is not caused by a disease of the mucous membrane of the middle ear, but rather by a primary disease of the otic capsule. This was the original description of otosclerosis! After attending the sessions of the Pan-American Congress, POLITZER visited the Mütter Museum where he noted that his specimens were in fine condition. – The state of preservation after the intervening decades is still good, and the collection can still be visited. The POLITZER collection reveals a variety of chronic changes involving the tympanic membranes and other temporal bone structures. Many of his anatomical preparations demonstrate the relationship of the tympanic membrane to the middle and inner ear structures in both children and adults; the topographical relationship of the semicircular canal and the cochlea to the drumhead; the occurrence of necrosis involving destruction of the conductive and sensory-neural structures with erosion into the sigmoid sinus; and the presence of semi-lunar, kidney-shaped, and multiple perforations of the tympanic membrane. For the otologist, a firsthand view of this historic collection at the Mütter Museum in Philadelphia is an educational inspiration. These specimens represent a tangible legacy which continues to be pertinent today.

POLITZER was regarded as a model teacher; not only was his knowledge profound, but he could inspire others with untiring zeal for conscientious work. His ability to teach with equal fluency in German, Hungarian, Bohemian, English, French, and Italian increased his popularity. He had only 4 pupils in his first course, but it was not long before students and otologists flocked to his clinic from all parts of the world. During his 46 years of active service, 7,000 physicians from all over the world participated in his courses in diseases of the ear. Erna LESKY points to the fact that POLITZER's very special teaching qualities not only resulted from his unique talent, but were "based on the broad foundation of a school where sickbed teaching had grown in a classic manner to a very characteristic art from DE HAEN to OPPOLZER; POLITZER related the success of his department to this teaching tradition of the Vienna school, and especially to the method handed down from his teachers OPPOLZER, SKODA, HEBRA, and ARLT."[44] He himself explained the roots of this success when he said: "It is this type of teaching, tied to direct observation of the patient, devoid of all superfluous theoretical accessories, which helps the student imprint on his memory the typical disease symptoms which he will later need as the foundation of his practical work. However, this method should in no way be seen as a mere unorganized description of cases, but on the contrary it is characterized by a critical analysis of the disease symptoms and processes based on exclusively scientific foundations, which stimulates the student to independent thinking and, in favorable circumstances, to research. With satisfaction we can state that the teaching

zudringen, daß der Arzt, soll sein Beruf voll erfaßt sein und nicht zum bloßen Handwerk herabgedrückt werden, den Entwicklungsgang seiner Wissenschaft, wenigstens in ihren Grundzügen, kennen muß"[50], sind heute noch genauso gültig wie damals, als POLITZER sie zu Papier brachte. Es hat freilich bis zum Jahr 1984 gedauert, daß seine Büste im Arkadenhof der Wiener Universität auf Anregung der Österreichischen Gesellschaft für Hals-, Nasen- und Ohrenheilkunde, Kopf- und Halschirurgie zwischen derjenigen von Clemens VON PIRQUET (1874–1929) und Richard Freiherrn VON KRAFFT-EBING (1840–1902) Aufstellung fand.

Bei seinem Überblick über die Leistungen der Ohrenheilkunde in Wien widmet POLITZER im zweiten Band seiner „Geschichte der Ohrenheilkunde" (Seiten 297 ff.) der Ohrenabteilung der Allgemeinen Poliklinik als einziger von allen damals in Wien bestehenden Ohrenabteilungen einen eigenen Abschnitt. Daß es sich dabei um keinen Zufall handelte, darauf hat Erna LESKY als erste hingewiesen[51], war doch die Allgemeine Poliklinik seit ihrer Gründung im Jahr 1872 „geradezu die Hochburg des Wiener Spezialistentums" (LESKY). Es ist hier nicht der Platz, eine Geschichte der Wiener Allgemeinen Poliklinik zu schreiben,[52] doch muß wenigstens in knapper Form auf diese Gründung, schon allein wegen ihrer außerordentlichen Stellung im medizinischen Leben Wiens, eingegangen werden.

Zu Jahresende 1871 erschien in der von Johann SCHNITZLER herausgegebenen ‚Wiener Medizinischen Presse' eine kurze Notiz „von der Poliklinik" mit dem Hinweis: „Am 2. Jänner kommenden Jahres wird die erste allgemeine Poliklinik in Wien eröffnet. Durch dieses neue Institut sollen nicht nur die Humanitätsanstalten der Residenz durch eine der wohlthätigsten bereichert, sondern wie wir hoffen, auch der praktisch-medizinische Unterricht nicht unwesentlich gefördert werden. Zweck der Anstalt ist unentgeltliche Ordination für unbemittelte Kranke durch bewährte Spezialisten, bei gleichzeitiger Verwerthung des Materials zu wissenschaftlichen und Lehrzwecken."[53] Der Grundgedanke für die Gründung der Poliklinik war also ein sozialer oder, wenn man will, humanitärer: in einem allgemeinen Ambulanzbetrieb sollte armen Kranken die Möglichkeit geboten sein, von qualifizierten Fachkräften unentgeltlich behandelt zu werden. Den jungen Dozenten – es waren zunächst zwölf, die in zwölf „Sectionen" oder Abteilungen ordinierten – bot sich aber gleichzeitig die Gelegenheit der freien wissenschaftlichen Forschung und eines eigenen Lehrbetriebes; konnten sie doch wegen der ständig steigenden Hörerfrequenz und den immer unleidlicher werdenden Platzverhältnissen auf den Kliniken und Instituten des Allgemeinen Krankenhauses nur unter größten Schwierigkeiten ihrer Lehrpflicht nachkommen. So bedeutete die Neugründung auch in wissenschaftlicher Hinsicht keine Konkurrenz, sondern eine Entlastung für die räumlich und personell beengten Verhältnisse an den Kliniken. Im Allgemeinen Krankenhaus und in den übrigen Spitälern Wiens bestanden auch damals schon Ambulatorien, die der breiten Masse der Bevölkerung zur Verfügung standen; neuartig war an der Poliklinik aber, daß nur habilitierte Fachärzte auf eigenes Risiko, ohne jede offizielle Subventionierung ein Institut schufen, das einerseits den Kranken Hilfe, den ordinierenden Ärzten aber die Möglichkeit bot, praktische Medizin zu lehren und sich in einzelnen Fachdisziplinen weiterzubilden und zu spezialisieren. Neben diesen klar als Grundidee aufscheinenden Prinzipien trat als förderndes Ele-

method of the Vienna School has also been adopted by various medical faculties in foreign countries."[45] To illustrate POLITZER's personality, his teaching methods and the circumstances at the Vienna clinics let us refer to the historical notes of one of these "7,000 physicians from all over the world."[45a] Alexander RANDALL was a graduate of St. John's College in Annapolis, Maryland, who then completed a three-year course in medicine at the University of Pennsylvania. In 1883, using funds from a legacy of his father, he went to Europe to further his studies. In Vienna he first worked in Ferdinand ARLT's (1812–1887) clinic, as the specialty field of ophthalmology was much more advanced in scientific and operative methods at the time than his later specialty, otology. His memoirs are filled with accounts of the difficulty in securing positions to study under a particular professor. In regard to Ottokar von CHIARI (1853–1918), for instance, he writes: "So though I had been told that he was the only man in Vienna who knew a nose when he saw one, I did not try for a course with him. . . . We learned little as to the nose diagnostically, and still less operatively, a bungling buff of galvano cautery of the posterior naries being only once attempted. Yet, neat larynx work with probe and forceps was often in evidence and probably an occasional tracheotomy, though I did not chance to see any. I got ZUCKERKANDLE's [Emil ZUCKERKANDL's] book ['Normale und pathologische Anatomie der Nasenhöhle und ihrer pneumatischen Anhänge' / 'Normal and Pathological Anatomy of the Nasal Cavity and its Pneumatic Appendices', Vienna, 1882] and took the first copy of it to Philadelphia and a few dozen temporals that I bought at 10 ¢ a piece, making the start of my collection." RANDALL then took a course in otology given by POLITZER: "His efficiency (sharp as a steel trap) showed us that an hour with POLITZER was worth at least a half a dozen of BINGS. With his mirror held by a handle between his teeth so as not to displace his scratch wig, he would spin around from one to another of his patients – 'Have you zeen?' With crayon and stamp he would dash off a crude sketch of drum head details, fasten it to the patient's shoulder and make his demonstration of the conditions to be observed, broaden the illustration by reference to pictures on the wall or specimens in his cabinet and enlarge upon the meaning and treatment. It was an admirable course on otoscopy with little or no stress on hearing tests or operative measures, for the Grippe Epidemics of slightly later years had not yet brought the numerous cases needing operation. One such did turn up and he showed it as needing a WILD's incision and had the assistants flying around here, there, and everywhere like headless chickens. Then, with little preparation and no anesthetic, he made his incision to the bone, fairly evacuating the pus, but opening a postauricular artery. Its spurt nearly washed him off his feet and utterly discombobulated him. Ligature and tenanculum were at hand, but hemostats were hardly yet known. He could not secure the spurter and would not let WOFFLER [WÖLFLER] do so when he had summoned him from BILLROTH's Klinic. So you can imagine the feelings of our group as WOFFLER took the man by the ear and marched him off to the quiet of his own clinic. It is notable that no other mastoid case appeared among the hundreds, even thousands, that came in those three months to the several clinics.

POLITZER and GRUBER, by the way, taught almost simultaneously in their wards – POLITZER in the women's and GRUBER in the men's, and each had one side of each adjoining room, so

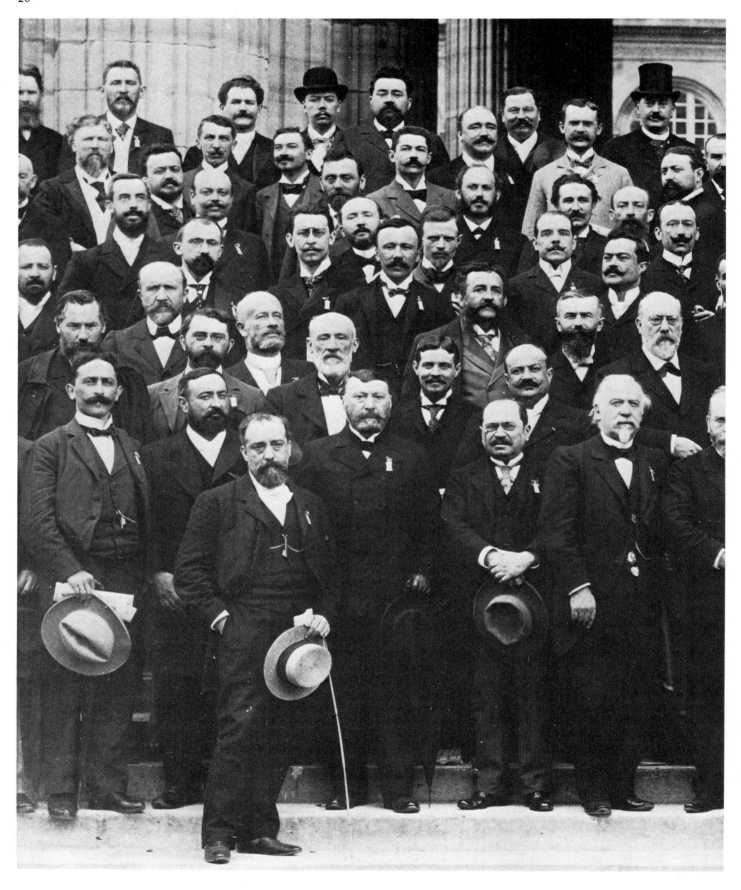

Links oben: Ernennungsurkunde für „Hofrath Prof. Adam Politzer" zum ersten Ehrenmitglied der American Medical Association of Vienna vom 1. Oktober 1907.

Top left: On October 1, 1907, "Hofrath Prof. Adam Politzer" was "unanimously declared the first honorary member" of the American Medical Association of Vienna. Depicted is the letter of appointment.

Links unten: Titelseite der englischen Übersetzung des ersten Bandes von Politzers „Geschichte der Ohrenheilkunde", die 1981 in den USA erschien.

Bottom left: Title page of the English translation of the first volume of Politzer's "Geschichte der Ohrenheilkunde" which appeared in the USA in 1981.

Rechts: Titelseite des zweiten Bandes von Politzers „Geschichte der Ohrenheilkunde" in Politzers Handschrift.

Right: Title page of the second volume of Politzer's "Geschichte der Ohrenheilkunde" in his own hand-writing.

Seite 28: Adam Politzer auf dem otolaryngologischen Kongreß in London im Jahr 1899.

Page 28: Adam Politzer at the Congress of Otolaryngology in London in 1899.

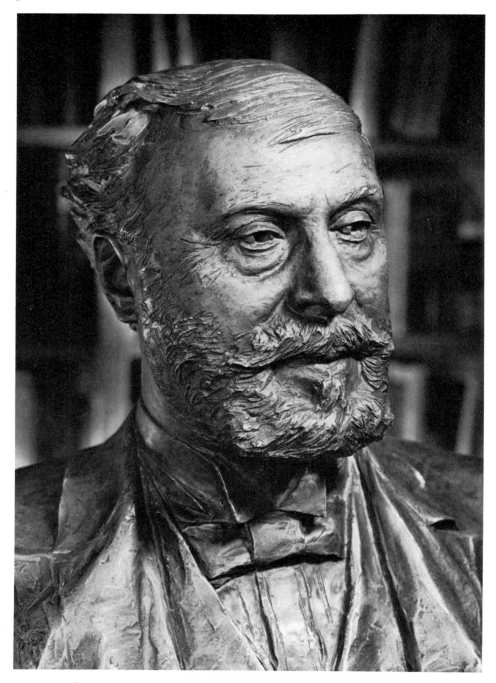

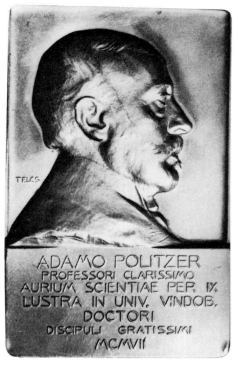

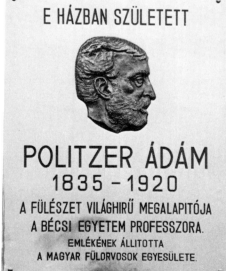

Bronzebüste Adam Politzers von Bernstamm, Paris, 1902. Im Besitz des Instituts für Geschichte der Medizin der Universität Wien.

Bronze bust of Adam Politzer by Bernstamm, Paris, 1902. In possession of the Institute for the History of Medicine of the University of Vienna.

Rechts oben: Dankplakette der Schüler für Adam Politzer aus dem Jahr 1907.

Top right: A commemorative plaque presented by Adam Politzer's students in 1907.

Rechts unten: Gedenktafel am Geburtshaus Politzers in Albertirsag (Alberti) in Ungarn, enthüllt 1973. Der Text lautet: „In diesem Haus wurde Adam Politzer (1835–1920), der weltberühmte Gründer der Otologie, Professor der Wiener Universität, geboren. Zur Erinnerung. Die Ungarische Oto-Laryngologische Gesellschaft."

Bottom right: Plaque at the birthplace of Politzer in Alberti, Hungary, unveiled in 1973, stating: "In this house Adam Politzer (1835–1920), the world famous founder of otology, Professor at the University of Vienna, was born. In his memory. The Hungarian Oto-Laryngological Society."

ment für die freie Forschung die Konzentration verschiedener Spitalzweige hervor. Diese Tatsache wirkte sich in der Entwicklung der Poliklinik überaus befruchtend auf die wissenschaftliche Arbeit aus. Ursprünglich auf ähnlichen Institutionen des Auslandes basierend, wurde die Wiener Poliklinik im Laufe der auf ihre Gründung folgenden zwei Jahrzehnte das Vorbild und Muster für gleichartige Gründungen in Budapest, Rom, Paris, Madrid, New York und anderen Städten der Vereinigten Staaten.

Die Gründungsversammlung fand in der Wohnung des späteren ersten Direktors der Poliklinik, Heinrich AUSPITZ (1835–1886), statt, und am 1. Jänner 1872 bezog die neugeschaffene Institution „einige kleine Zimmerchen in dem dunklen Hofraume eines alten Hauses in der Wipplingerstrasse",[54] wie sich Johann SCHNITZLER 1884 erinnert. Drei Jahre danach, „das anfangs unansehnliche und unbeachtete Institut entwickelte sich allmälig, aber stetig"[55], übersiedelte die inzwischen offiziell als Verein anerkannte Poliklinik in eine Seitengasse der Mölkerbastei, Ecke Franzensring. Über Vorschlag der Poliklinik erhielt die Gasse den Namen Oppolzergasse. Im Jahr 1879 übersiedelte dann die Poliklinik in einen Neubau, Schwarzspanierstraße 12, wo sie eingemietet über zehn Jahre verblieb. War die Finanzierung zunächst Privatsache der zwölf Gründungsmitglieder, so gelang es, großzügige Spenden – etwa von Fürstin Pauline METTERNICH oder vom Protektor der Anstalt, Erzherzog RAINER – zu erhalten, wodurch 1891 ein Grundstück in der Mariannengasse 10, in unmittelbarer Nachbarschaft der Universitäts-Kliniken, angekauft werden konnte. Hier entstand in den Jahren 1891/92 der Neubau der Allgemeinen Poliklinik. Im November 1944 wurde die Poliklinik durch einen Bombenangriff so schwer beschädigt, daß das Haus Mariannengasse 12 von offizieller Seite her gesperrt werden mußte. Trotzdem begann die Ärzteschaft mit dem Pflegepersonal sofort mit den Aufräumungsarbeiten und bald konnte wieder ein Ambulanzbetrieb aufgenommen und die Adaptierung der Abteilungen begonnen werden.

Schon im ersten Jahr ihres Bestehens berichtete die ‚Wiener Medizinische Presse' „von der allgemeinen Poliklinik": „Die Poliklinik gewinnt immer mehr Sympathien im Publikum, und wie wir mit besonderer Befriedigung bemerken, allmälig auch anerkennende Würdigung von Seite der Aerzte. Diese scheinen zur Ueberzeugung gelangt zu sein, dass die Gründer der Poliklinik keinen anderen Zweck verfolgen, als sich in ihrer Eigenschaft als Universitätsdocenten selbständiges Material für wissenschaftliche und Unterrichtszwecke zu verschaffen, und dies ist ihnen auch in einem alle Erwartung übersteigenden Masse gelungen. . . . In letzterer Zeit sind dem Verband der Poliklinik auch einige neue Kräfte beigetreten; so Prof. LEIDESDORF, der über Gehirn- und Nervenkrankheiten, Dozent Dr. MONTI, der über Kinderkrankheiten lesen, und Dr. URBANTSCHITSCH, der für Ohrenkranke ordiniren wird."[56]

Viktor URBANTSCHITSCH (1847–1921) war damals 25 Jahre alt, zwei Jahre promoviert (1870) und gerade erst (1872) mit einer Arbeit „Beiträge zur Embryologie des Ohres" habilitiert, als ihn Wilhelm WINTERNITZ (1843–1917) im Jahr 1872 als Vorstand für die neuerrichtete Ohrenabteilung der Poliklinik vorschlug. So entstand bereits ein Jahr *vor* der Gründung der Universitäts-Ohrenklinik eine eigene Ohrenabteilung an der Poliklinik! WINTERNITZ, der „geistige Initiator der Allgemeinen Poliklinik",[57] hatte URBANTSCHITSCH den Rat gege-

when POLITZER spoke rather contemptuously of a certain Joseph GRUBER and the latter in the like manner of POLITZER, it was before a row of the other man's patients and with WIETHE often present as an assistant to each. WIETHE was supposed to be an oculist as well as an aurist and ought to have had a little dexterity, but he usually succeeded in making the nose bleed every time he did a POLITZER inflation. So I should credit him with having six thumbs instead of the five commonly on each German hand. I should have liked to study with GRUBER, but with my work occupying most of my time, I could hardly manage both and was too well pleased with POLITZER's teaching to change from him, especially when in more intimate relation with him over the photographic work." RANDALL procured a small camera and an appropriate lens and so described his further relationship with POLITZER: "When POLITZER started his teaching in the fall, I coveted pictures of the specimen he showed us. POLITZER assented joyously. He had tried photography himself but with little success, as he had fallen far short of ULTZMAN's [ULTZMANN's] solar pictures. That we could work without elaborate heilostat at night and a tiny oil lamp delighted him. Many an evening he came to my room bringing some of his choice specimens for MORRIS and me to try out. When we departed, he gave each of us quite a valuable series of slides. Our photographs, poor, but neatly mounted, he framed and hung up on his clinic walls, and it was 'no small feather in my cap' when men returning would say, 'I saw your photographs framed on POLITZER's wall.' It was a start from which MORRIS and I built up photographic illustrations of the anatomy of the ear that was to help the election for each of us to the American Otologic Society a little later, and to my call to the Professorship at Poly Clinic in '88 and the University of Pennsylvania in '91. My old Housefrau was greatly stirred by the presence with us in her room of Herr Professor Dr. POLITZER, but fortunately did not suffer her expected stroke of apoplexy until the following summer after we had left." After GRUBER's retirement in 1897, POLITZER became the sole chief of the Clinic of Otology and after the clinic was expanded, he held his inaugural address on the duties concerning the instruction of otology. In this address POLITZER expressed his hope that "from now on instruction in otiatry, which despite its meager facilities at the University of Vienna did not have to be afraid of comparison with foreign well-equipped otiatric clinics, can now be given in such a way that is comparable to the high esteem of our university. Thus, the sick-rooms of the clinic of otology may be used as they should be and will not be affected by the turmoil in the out-patient departments any longer."[46] – At that time the out-patients numbered 15,000 per year and the number of mastoidectomies and radical operations was 400.[47]

In 1907, when he reached the age of 70, POLITZER had to retire. At the German Congress of Otologists in 1906, he gave a report on the position of otology: "We can only point to those otological procedures which can be considered amongst the most difficult techniques in modern surgery. I particularly have in mind the surgical therapy of otogenic brain abscesses and thrombosis of the intracranial sinuses. These operations have enabled interventions on many patients who had previously been considered hopeless."[48]

POLITZER trained an immense number of students and physicians from all over the world; his clinic was a true 'Mecca' for

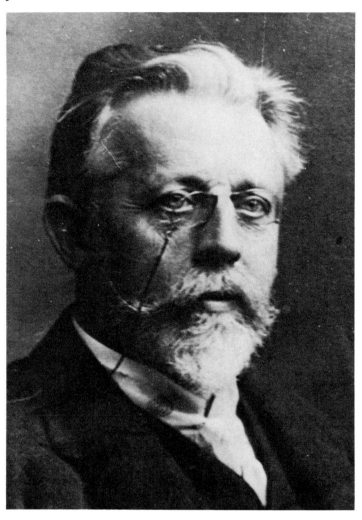

Viktor von Urbantschitsch

ben, otologische Kurse bei Politzer und Gruber zu besuchen, aber dort nicht mitzuteilen, daß er als Ohrenarzt für die Poliklinik vorgesehen sei. Es ist erstaunlich, blickt man auf sein Œvre, wie sich Urbantschitsch zum größten Teil autodidaktisch in das ganze Gebiet der Ohrenheilkunde einarbeitete. Zum Zeitpunkt seiner Berufung an die Poliklinik lagen von ihm sechs Arbeiten vor; im Jahr 1918 hält sein Arbeitenverzeichnis[58] bei der Zahl siebenundsechzig. Eine seiner ersten Arbeiten war ein Beitrag zur Schallperzeption, an die sich dann eine Reihe von Veröffentlichungen über otologische Akustik anschlossen. Urbantschitschs Forschungen über die Anatomie der Ohrtrompete bilden die Grundlage für die therapeutische Beeinflussung der Tube und des Mittelohres. Seine im Jahr 1883 erschienene Arbeit „Über die Bougierung der Ohrtrompete" leitete einen neuen Abschnitt der Therapie ein. Seinem menschlichen und ärztlichen Empfinden folgend – bei seiner Antrittsrede anläßlich der Übernahme der Universitäts-Ohrenklinik im Jahr 1907 sagte er u. a.: „Was ... die Schwerhörigkeit betrifft, so bildet diese eine der meist verbreiteten Krankheitserscheinungen, die je nach ihrem Grade und dem Lebensalter, in der sie auftritt, das Lebensglück der davon Betroffenen mehr oder weniger tief zu schädigen vermag"[59] – beschäftigte er sich sowohl mit der Behandlung der hochgradigen Schwerhörigkeit als auch der Fürsorge

otologists. With his scientific work, Politzer erected an everlasting monument, and he was far ahead of all his contemporaries in promoting a permanent expansion of otology. During his 46 years of teaching, Politzer turned otology from a "sterile, hopeless discipline" into an academically recognized specialty. In 1864, Politzer, together with Anton Friedrich von Tröltsch (1829–1890) and Hermann Schwartze (1837–1910), founded the "Archives of Otology". In 1895, in association with Josef Gruber and Viktor von Urbantschitsch (1847–1921), he founded the Austrian Otological Society.

Politzer's methods and research have been passed on in turn from his 'children', his closest students and co-workers, to their students, thus forming a living chain whose gratitude has immortalized him and his work. With deep satisfaction he stated at the end of his academic career: "It fills my heart both with pride and joy that most of the assistants who stood at my side at the beginning of my career as academic teacher have become academic teachers themselves."[49] Few men have left such a rich heritage of outstanding assistants whom they have trained and who made such memorable contributions to the field of oto-laryngology, especially otology. There was a Politzer School, and at the following Viennese hospitals out-patient departments for otology or departments of oto-

Gustav Alexander

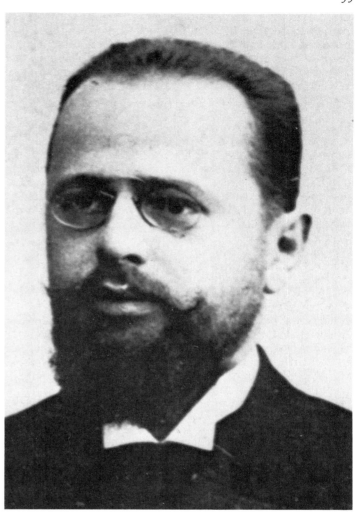

für Spätertaubte und Taubstumme. Die Aufdeckung von Hörresten nach seiner Methode mit der Harmonika an Stelle der Stimmgabel, seine Methode der Wiedererziehung des Gehörs Ertaubter durch methodische Hörübungen eroberte bald die ganze Welt und fand besonders in Frankreich und Amerika Nachahmung. Es ist auch das Verdienst URBANT-SCHITSCHS, den elektrischen Strom in jeder Form in die Therapie eingeführt zu haben. „Wenn auch diese Behandlungsmethode nur manchesmal von Erfolg begleitet ist, so ist sie doch bei der Behandlung von unheilbaren Ohrenerkrankungen, wie Otosklerose und Labyrintherkrankung, schon mit Rücksicht auf die Psyche des Patienten unentbehrlich. Wahrlich es gehört der Mut der ehrlichen Überzeugung dazu, eine so vielfach angefeindete Behandlungsmethode zu empfehlen und zu vertreten; aber die rasche Verbreitung derselben gab URBANTSCHITSCH recht", schreibt Heinrich NEUMANN im Nachruf auf URBANTSCHITSCH.[60] Eine ganze Reihe von Behandlungsmethoden und Apparaten sind auf Grund von URBANTSCHITSCHS Angaben zustande gekommen und in die ohrenärztliche Praxis übernommen worden. URBANTSCHITSCH entwickelte an der Poliklinik eine rege praktische und wissenschaftliche Tätigkeit, hielt regelmäßig otologische Vorlesungen für Studierende und Ärzte, u. a. auch Kurse über den Einfluß methodischer Hörübungen auf den Hör-

logy were established during POLITZER's life: in 1892, Benjamin GOMPERZ (1861–1935) became head of the Department of Otology of the First Public Institute for Sick Children. He published among other monographs a work on "Pathology and Therapy of Otitis Media in Infancy" (Vienna, 1906). In the period 1898–1908 Daniel KAUFMANN (1864–1919) worked as head of the Department of Otology of the Kaiser Franz-Josef Hospital. This department was taken over in 1909 by Hugo FREY (1873–1951), and in 1912 bei Heinrich NEUMANN (1873–1939), who had trained under POLITZER from 1900 to 1907, and who himself in 1919 became head of the Clinic of Otology. Ferdinand ALT (1867–1923) founded out-patient departments for otological patients at the Rudolf's Hospital and the Wieden Hospital in 1900; he displayed a special interest in occupational damage to the auditory organ. POLITZER was not only the founder of the specialty in Vienna, he remains to this day also its historian thanks to his "History of Otology". The following sentences from the 'Foreword' are still valid today: "The history of medicine has long been neglected. Toward the end of the nineteenth century an increased interest in history as a whole became manifest. This historical trend, however, has only recently been reflected in the field of medicine. It has become increasingly evident to the physician that in order to gain a thorough understanding

sinn, die sich alle eines regen Zustromes, auch aus dem Ausland, erfreuten. Er befaßte sich auch mit psychophysiologischen Themen auf dem Gebiete der Ohrenerkrankungen; seine diesbezüglichen Arbeiten sind ein markantes Bindeglied zwischen Psychologie und Otologie.

1892 übersiedelte URBANTSCHITSCH mit der Poliklinik aus dem Haus in der Schwarzspanierstraße 12 im IX. Wiener Gemeindebezirk in das neue Heim in die Mariannengasse 10, im selben Bezirk, wo er zusammen mit Johann SCHNITZLER in den gleichen Räumen arbeitete. Nach GRUBERS Tod übernahm URBANTSCHITSCH die Herausgabe der Monatsschrift für Ohrenheilkunde, in seinen wissenschaftlichen Bestrebungen durch seinen Sohn Ernst v. URBANTSCHITSCH (1877–1948) unterstützt. Als Assistenten arbeiteten bei URBANTSCHITSCH an der Poliklinik u. a. Gustav BONDY (1870–1954), Bernhard PANZER, Maximilian RAUCH und Conrad STEIN (1870–1940). Bereits 1880 erschien URBANTSCHITSCHS „Lehrbuch der Ohrenheilkunde", das bis 1910 in fünf Auflagen gedruckt wurde. Drei Jahre vorher, 1907, wurde URBANTSCHITSCH, der bereits 1885 zum außerordentlichen Professor ernannt worden war, als Nachfolger POLITZERS mit der Leitung der Wiener Ohrenklinik betraut.

Nachfolger von URBANTSCHITSCH an der Ohrenabteilung der Allgemeinen Poliklinik wurde 1907 der POLITZER-Schüler Gustav ALEXANDER (1873–1932; Dr. med. 1898, Dozent 1903, Titular-Extraordinarius 1909, Titular-Professor 1919).[61] Die gründliche Ausbildung, die ALEXANDER unter seinen Lehrern, dem Anatomen Emil ZUCKERKANDL (1849–1910), dem Chirurgen Eduard ALBERT (1841–1900) und Adam POLITZER genossen hatte, bildete die Basis seines weiteren klinischen Arbeitens. ALEXANDERS Arbeitsgebiet – aus seiner Hand stammen über 200 wissenschaftliche Arbeiten – umfaßt vor allem vier große Themen: Anatomie, Physiologie, pathologische Anatomie des Gehörorganes und die Klinik der Ohrenkrankheiten, vor allem die intrakraniellen Komplikationen.

Auf Grund seiner grundlegenden Kenntnisse war ALEXANDER ein Meister der klinischen Ohrenheilkunde. Das Lieblingsgebiet seiner Forschungen war die Ohr-Chirurgie mit besonderer Berücksichtigung der Diagnose und Therapie der otogenen Sinusthrombose; er gab auch eine Operationsmethode zum Verschluß retroaurikulärer Fisteln an, eine plastische Methode bei Mißbildungen der Ohrmuschel und eine Operationsmethode zur transauralen Operation der Akustikus-Tumoren. ALEXANDER prägte den Begriff „Mastoidismus" und war ein ausgesprochener Gegner der „Früh"-Operation bei Mastoiditis, womit er sich in Gegensatz zu vielen anderen Autoren setzte. 1906 hat er in ALBERTS Lehrbuch der Chirurgie das Kapitel über die Chirurgie der Erkrankungen des Ohres verfaßt, gab 1912 das instruktive Lehrbuch der „Ohrenkrankheiten des Kindesalters" heraus und 1925 mit J. FISCHER eine „Präparationstechnik des Gehörorgans". Im Handbuch der HNO-Krankheiten von DENKER-KAHLER bearbeitete ALEXANDER 1926 die Abschnitte „Entwicklungsgeschichte, Anthropologie, Varietäten" und „Die nicht eitrigen Erkrankungen des Innenohres, Innenohraffektion und allgemeine Erkrankung". Mit Otto MARBURG (1874–1948) gab ALEXANDER 1926 das dreibändige Handbuch der „Neurologie des Ohres" heraus.

Außer den wissenschaftlichen Themen befaßte sich ALEXANDER mit Vorliebe auch mit sozialen. Sein reges Interesse dafür bewies er schon durch seine Tätigkeit als Schulohrenarzt in

of medicine he must have at least a rudimentary knowledge of its developmental history."[50]. POLITZER retained his keen interest in otology to the very end of his days. At the age of 84, Adolf KRONFELD, the editor of the "Vienna Medical Weekly" described him as having delivered a historical review at the 25th anniversary of the Austrian Otological Society (March 29, 1920) "extemporaneously with his usual spiritual and bodily vigor". It was on this occasion that POLITZER said: "Regardless of the sad state into which our country has sunk due to the war, it is the duty of all who have at heart the advance of science, to look undismayed into the future, and with all the forces to assume the interrupted work. Upon you, my younger colleagues, does this duty rest. It requires now, more than ever, devotion, industry and perseverance. Your are confronted with more difficult tasks than we, your elders had in former days (although not without struggles), when it was granted us in quiet times to consecrate ourselves to scientific pursuits."[50a] – It was only in 1984 that POLITZER's bust was unveiled in the Arcades of the University of Vienna. It is not by chance, as Erna LESKY points out,[51] that POLITZER devoted a special chapter to the Otology Department of the General Policlinic when summing up the achievements of otology in Vienna in the second volume of his "History of Otology". The General Policlinic had been "the focus of specialization in Vienna"[52] from its establishment in 1872. Let us briefly sketch the founding of the Policlinic: At the end of 1871 a short note appeared in Johann SCHNITZLER's "Vienna Medical Press" which read: "On January 2, 1872, the General Policlinic, the first of its kind in Vienna, will be opened. The new institution will not only help to ease the burden of overcrowded hospitals in Vienna but also provide practical medical education."[53] The basic idea, therefore, in founding the Policlinic was, on the one hand, to offer free medical help to the indigent section of the population of Vienna and, on the other hand, to establish an additional medical teaching institution apart from the General Hospital. In the General Hospital the wards were crowded and it became more and more difficult if not impossible for young lecturers to find sufficient opportunities for continuing their research. A group of twelve young lecturers under the leadership of Heinrich AUSPITZ (1835–1886) took the initiative and provided their own teaching material by opening a policlinic – an out-patient department – on Wipplingerstrasse in 1872. It was new that only lecturers who were also specialists in their fields were allowed to practice at the Policlinic (out-patient departments already existed in the General Hospital and in other Viennese hospitals). Besides, the Policlinic was a solely private institution without any public funding. This was indeed a praiseworthy attempt; however, especially the fact that poor people were treated there free-of-charge was regarded as a threat to their private practice by the physicians of Vienna. For many years complaints and accusations appeared in medical journals against these very active and capable policlinicians. The public, however, liked the new institution: soon it was able to move from its old home "where it occupied a few small rooms in the back side of an old house in Wipplingerstrasse"[54] to a more suitable location, because the institution grew "gradually but steadily"[55]. In 1879 the Policlinic moved to a new house in Schwarzspanier Strasse where it remained for more than ten years. In 1891 a site was purchased – with the help of the tireless Duchess Pauline METTERNICH and the patron of the Policlinic, Archduke Rainer – in Mariannengasse, next to

Berndorf. Gerade das Taubstummenwesen hatte für ihn von jeher eine besondere Anziehungskraft. Seine Bemühungen trugen wesentlich zur Schaffung des ersten Taubstummen-Kindergartens in Österreich (1916) bei. In gleicher Weise setzte sich ALEXANDER für die Taubstummblinden ein, deren kleines Heim in Wien-Hietzing er sein besonderes Augenmerk zuwendete.

ALEXANDER gab zahlreiche Instrumente an, u. a. die nach ihm benannte Ohrspritze; er führte den langen Hohlmeißel ein und eine Reihe anderer Spezialinstrumente. Ihm ist auch die Modernisierung des otologischen Operationsbetriebes zu danken; war er doch der erste, der anstelle der „Billroth-Schürze" und der Operation mit aufgesteckten Hemdsärmeln ein richtiges Operationsteam mit Assistenten und Operationsschwester und sterilen Operationsmänteln einführte. Auf eigene Kosten richtete ALEXANDER ein mit den modernsten Behelfen ausgestattetes histologisches Laboratorium ein, aus dem die meisten seiner wissenschaftlichen Arbeiten und die seiner Schüler hervorgingen. Seine Assistenten waren u. a.: Oskar BENESI, Hans BRUNNER, Alexander CEMACH, Josef FISCHER, Rudolf LEIDLER, Josef SCHMIERER, Ignatz SOMMER und Leopold STEIN.

In das erste Jahrzehnt unseres Jahrhunderts fallen die epochemachenden Entwicklungen auf dem Gebiet der 1914 mit dem Nobelpreis gekrönten Wiener Vestibularisforschung.[62] Bereits in einer seiner ersten, gemeinsam mit Gustav ALEXANDER veröffentlichten Arbeiten beschäftigte sich Robert BÁRÁNY (1876–1936; Dr. med. 1900, Dozent 1909, o. Prof. [Uppsala] 1926) mit der Bedeutung des Gleichgewichtsapparates für die Orientierung im Raum bei Gesunden und Taubstummen. Seine Untersuchungsmethoden und Forschungen über die Funktion des Gleichgewichtsapparates sind gerade in der jüngsten Gegenwart, im Zeitalter der Weltraumfahrt, von besonderer Aktualität.

Lange Zeit hatte man vom Gleichgewichts-(Vestibular-)Apparat nur eine Art ‚mystische' Vorstellung. Zwar hatte sich bereits 1820 der Prager Physiologieprofessor J. E. PURKINJE mit Untersuchungen über den Schwindel auf Grund von Selbstversuchen beschäftigt. Es war auch bereits seit langem bekannt, daß im Innenohr drei senkrecht zueinander angeordnete, halbzirkelförmige Kanäle, die Bogengänge, vorhanden sind. Nach Durchschneidung der Bogengänge bei Tauben durch M. J. P. FLOURENS (1824) in Straßburg traten Kopfbewegungen und Körperdrehungen und auch heftige Augenbewegungen (Nystagmus) auf. 1861 beschrieb der Pariser Arzt P. MENIÈRE eine mit schweren Schwindelanfällen, Erbrechen und Schwerhörigkeit einhergehende Erkrankung, als deren Ursache er bei einem tödlich verlaufenen Fall Veränderungen in den Bogengängen feststellte. 1874 teilten dann unabhängig voneinander der praktische Arzt Josef BREUER aus Wien, der Edinburger Chemiker A. CRUM BROWN und der Wiener Physiker Ernst MACH ihre zum Teil tierexperimentellen Untersuchungsergebnisse mit[63], und zwar, daß der Gleichgewichtsapparat aus zwei Sinnesorganen bestehe, von denen die Vorhofsäckchen mit den Otolithen für die Empfindung der Lage im Raum und für geradlinige Beschleunigungen verantwortlich seien, während die drei Bogengänge die Empfindung von Drehbewegungen vermittelten. MACH und BREUER nahmen als auslösende Ursache der beschriebenen Erscheinungen eine Strömung der in den Bogengängen enthaltenen Flüssigkeit, der Endolymphe, an. Es fehlte jedoch der Beweis, daß die im Tierexperiment erhaltenen Ergebnisse auch auf den

the Clinics of the University. Here the new Policlinic was erected in 1891/92. In 1944 this building was heavily bombed and damaged, but due to the initiative of the practicing physicians, nurses and other staff the out-patient departments could be re-opened and before long the reconstruction began.

Already in the first year of its existence the "Vienna Medical Press" reported: "The popularity of the Policlinic is steadily growing and even the physicians seem to accept its existence. Lately the staff of the Policlinic was joined by new members: Prof. LEIDESDORF, who will do practice in brain- and nerve diseases, Docent Dr. MONTI, who will lecture in pediatrics, and Dr. URBANTSCHITSCH, who will practice otology."[56] Viktor URBANTSCHITSCH (1847–1921), son of a Viennese physician, was only 25 years old in 1872, had graduated two years previously, and had just been appointed lecturer in otology (1872) when he was proposed by Wilhelm WINTERNITZ (1843–1917) to become head of the newly established otology department at the Policlinic. Thus, the General Policlinic had its Department of Otology one year *prior* to the Department of Otology at the University of Vienna! WINTERNITZ, "one of the spiritual initiators of the General Policlinic"[57], had suggested to URBANTSCHITSCH to attend courses in otology under POLITZER and GRUBER, but not to tell them that he was to become otologist at the Policlinic. It is remarkable to note how quickly URBANTSCHITSCH mastered the whole field of otology by teaching himself the subject.

At the time URBANTSCHITSCH became head of the Department of Otology at the Policlinic he had six publications to his name; in 1918 his publications numbered 67.[58] One of his early works was on the perception of sound, which was followed by a number of other publications concerning the physiology of acoustics. His research on the anatomy of the auditory tube formed the basis for the treatment of diseases of the Eustachian tube and the middle ear. With his publication "On the Bouginage of the Auditory Tube" (1883), a new era in therapy began. In 1893 URBANTSCHITSCH took up the problem of deaf-mutism.

In 1907 URBANTSCHITSCH succeeded POLITZER as head of the University Clinic of Otology. In his inaugural lecture he said: "Deaf-mutism is one of the most common diseases, which has an enormously negative effect on the quality of the life of those who are affected."[59] According to his thesis – deaf-mutism being due to lethargy and inactivity of the auditory nerve, and that this nerve might be activated by hearing exercises – URBANTSCHITSCH tried to activate the hearing power of deaf-mutes by methodical exercises, by having them repeat single letters, sounds and short sentences after these had been phonated by the physician. In doing so he met with strong criticism from his professional colleagues, especially when using electricity therapeutically. "Truly, one would need the courage of honest convictions to recommend and represent a teaching method which has met with so much animosity", Heinrich NEUMANN said, adding, however, "but rapid acceptance put URBANTSCHITSCH in the right."[60] His methods soon became popular not only in Austria but also in France and the United States. Around the turn of the century URBANTSCHITSCH's department at the Policlinic was the Mecca of deaf-mutes. He became the father of audiology and his research on the psycho-physiology of otology linked psychology with otology.

In 1892 his department at the Policlinic moved to new prem-

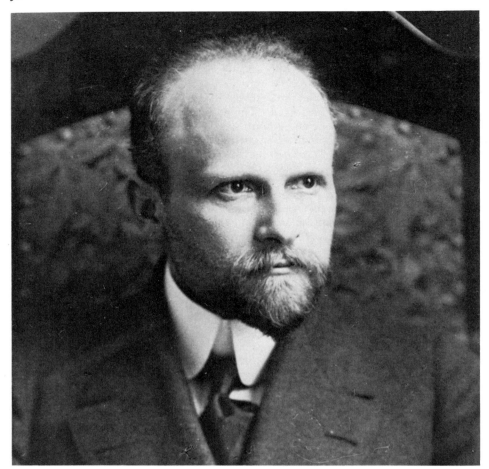

Links: Der Nobelpreisträger Robert Bárány. Bárány erhielt 1914 den Nobelpreis für Physiologie und Medizin „für seine Arbeiten über die Physiologie und Pathologie des Vestibularisapparates".
Seite 37 oben: Lärmtrommel nach Bárány zur Prüfung einseitiger Taubheit.

Left: The Nobel Prize winner Robert Bárány. In 1914 Robert Bárány was awarded the Nobel Prize in Physiology and Medicine "for his work on the physiology and pathology of the vestibular apparatus."
Page 37 top: Bárány's noise-box.

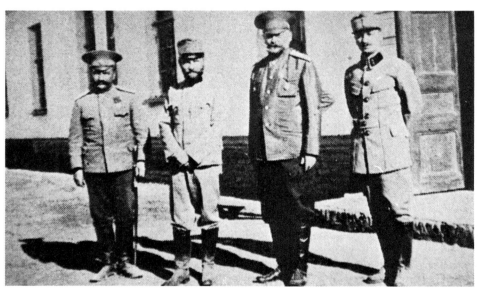

Unten: Robert Bárány in russischer Kriegsgefangenschaft in Merv, wo er 1915 die Nachricht von der Verleihung des Nobelpreises erhielt. Sein Danktelegramm an Professor Gunnar Holmgren in Stockholm ist unterschrieben „dr barany kriegsgefangener".

Bottom: When Robert Bárány was awarded the Nobel Prize for his research on the vestibular organ, he was a Russian prisoner of war in Merv (Turkestan). From there he sent a telegram to Prof. Gunnar Holmgren in Stockholm thanking him for the great honour, which he signed "dr barany, prisoner of war."

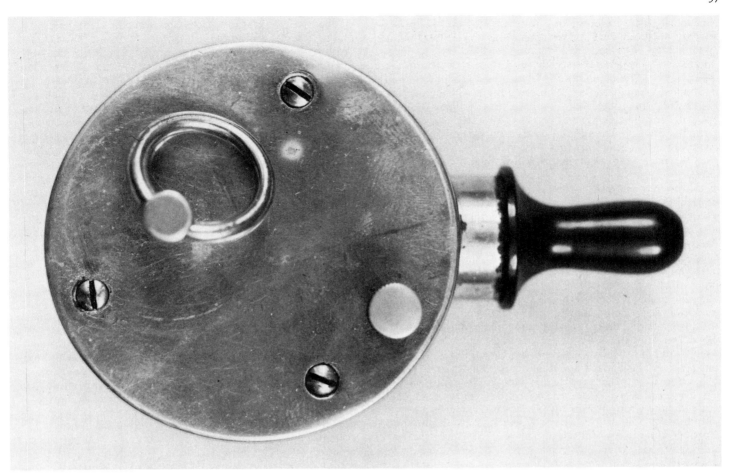

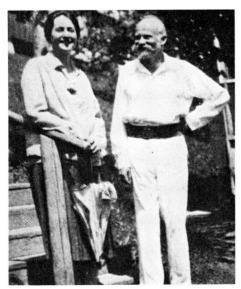

Links unten: Bárány mit Gattin in Uppsala (Schweden), wohin er 1917 eine Berufung an die Ohrenklinik annahm. 1926 wurde er ordentlicher Professor für Ohren-Nasen-Hals-Heilkunde an der Universität in Uppsala.

Bottom left: Bárány with his wife in Uppsala (Sweden). In 1917 Bárány received a call to the clinic of otology there, and in 1926 he became full professor of ENT-diseases at the University of Uppsala.

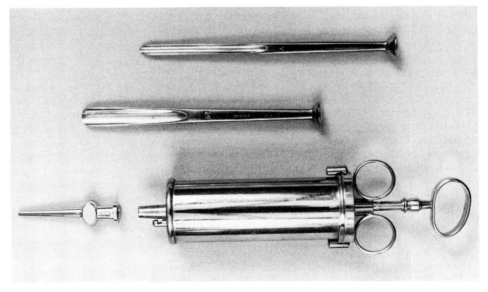

Rechts unten: Alexander-Meissel. Alexander-Spritze mit Bajonettverschluß.

Bottom right: Alexander-chisel. Alexander-syringe with bayonet fitting.

Menschen angewendet werden könnten. Vor allem fehlte es an einer Methode der Funktionsprüfung des Gleichgewichtsapparates am Menschen. Hier nun setzten die Forschungen und in der Folge Entdeckungen von Robert BÁRÁNY ein, über deren Geschichte er in seinem Vortrag am 11. September 1916 in Stockholm anläßlich der Überreichung des Nobelpreises für Physiologie und Medizin – es war dies der Preis des Jahres 1914, der infolge des Krieges erst 1915 BÁRÁNY „für seine Arbeiten über die Physiologie und Pathologie des Vestibularisapparates" zuerkannt wurde – berichtet: „Ich war als junger Ohrenarzt an der Klinik des Hofrat Prof. POLITZER [BÁRÁNY trat am 1. Oktober 1903 in die Klinik ein; am 7. Oktober 1905 wurde er noch unter POLITZER Assistent an der Klinik] in Wien tätig. Unter meinen Patienten befanden sich viele, bei denen ich eine Ausspülung des Ohres vornehmen mußte. Eine Anzahl dieser Patienten klagte nach dem Ausspülen über Schwindel. Es lag nahe für mich, ihre Augen anzusehen, und da bemerkte ich einen Augennystagmus von bestimmter Richtung. Ich notierte mir die Beobachtung. Nach einiger Zeit, als ich zirka 20 Beobachtungen gesammelt hatte, verglich ich sie untereinander und war überrascht, überall dieselbe Beobachtung verzeichnet zu finden. Da erkannte ich, daß diesen Beobachtungen ein allgemeines Gesetz zugrunde liegen muß. Doch wußte ich noch nicht, welches der Grund der Gesetzmäßigkeit sei. Ein Zufall kam mir zu Hilfe. Einer der Patienten, den ich ausspritzte, erklärte mir: ‚Herr Doktor, ich werde nur dann schwindelig, wenn das Wasser nicht warm genug ist. Wenn ich mich zu Hause ausspüle und genug warmes Wasser benütze, werde ich nicht schwindelig.' Darauf rief ich die Wärterin und gab ihr den Auftrag, mir zur Ausspülung wärmeres Wasser zu reichen. Sie erklärte, das Wasser sei warm genug. Ich erwiderte, wenn der Patient es als zu kalt empfindet, müssen wir uns nach dem Patienten richten. Das nächste Mal gab sie nun sehr heißes Wasser in den Ballon. Als ich den Patienten ausspülte, rief er aus: ‚Aber Herr Doktor, das Wasser ist viel zu heiß, jetzt werde ich wieder schwindelig.' Rasch beobachtete ich die Augen des Patienten und bemerkte, daß jetzt der Augennystagmus genau umgekehrt gerichtet war als früher bei Ausspülung mit zu kaltem Wasser."[64] – Dadurch hatte BÁRÁNY erstmalig die Gesetzmäßigkeit des „kalorischen Nystagmus", d. h. der Augenzuckungen, die durch Differenzen der Wassertemperatur (im Vergleich zur Körpertemperatur) bei Ohrspülungen auftreten, nachgewiesen. So wurde von BÁRÁNY die Grundlage seiner späteren Lehre von der Physiologie und Pathologie des menschlichen Gleichgewichtsapparates geschaffen. Durch diese Prüfmethode war es zum ersten Mal auch möglich, das Innenohr beiderseits getrennt auf die Funktionsfähigkeit der Gleichgewichtsapparate zu untersuchen und so eine Klinik der verschiedenen Innenohrerkrankungen aufzustellen.
Neben der Spülmethode mit verschiedengradigem Wasser verwendete BÁRÁNY auch die Drehprüfung zur Untersuchung des Gleichgewichtsapparates. Ausgehend von der MACH-BREUER'schen Endolymphströmungstheorie im Bogengang konstruierte er aus einem Untersuchungsstockerl der Klinik einen einfachen Drehstuhl. Bei der so durchgeführten Drehprüfung konnte er beobachten, daß es während der Drehung zu rhythmischen Augenzuckungen in der Drehrichtung, nach plötzlichem Anhalten zu einem ruckartigen Augenzucken (Nystagmus) entgegengesetzt zur Drehrichtung kommt. Die isolierte Vestibularausschaltung beschrieb er erstmals 1907, in

ises in Vienna's ninth district, Mariannengasse. Here URBANTSCHITSCH shared the rooms with Johann SCHNITZLER. Among URBANTSCHITSCH's assistants at the Policlinic were Gustav BONDY (1870–1954), Bernhard PANZER, Maximilian RAUCH, Conrad STEIN (1870–1940). In 1880 URBANTSCHITSCH published his "Textbook of Otology", which covered the subject exhaustively. In 1910, the fifth edition of this work appeared. Three years earlier, in 1907, URBANTSCHITSCH had succeeded POLITZER as head of the University Clinic of Otology, where he remained until 1917. With his noble and conciliatory character he was able to lessen the many tensions among the Viennese otologists. The Austrian Otological Society, of which he was a co-founder with POLITZER and GRUBER, was especially grateful to him for this achievement.
URBANTSCHITSCH was followed in the Policlinic's Department of Otology by Gustav ALEXANDER (1873–1932; M.D. 1898, lecturer 1903, "titular" associate professor 1909, "titular" full professor 1919).[61] The thorough training he had received under his teachers, the anatomist Emil ZUCKERKANDL (1849–1910), the surgeon Eduard ALBERT (1841–1900), and Adam POLITZER became the basis of his clinical work. ALEXANDER's impressive scientific work – all in all more than 200 publications – center on research in anatomy, physiology, and pathological anatomy of the auditory organ, and clinic of ear diseases, especially of intra-cranial complications. His preferred field of research was otological surgery with special emphasis on diagnosis and therapy of otological sinus thrombosis. His research of the labyrinth and the vestibular nerve already belongs to the 20th century. He coined the term "mastoidism", and opposed "early" mastoiditis operations. He contributed the chapter on surgery of otologic diseases to ALBERT's "Textbook of Surgery" and in 1912 he published the instructive "Textbook of Children's Diseases of the Ear".
Apart from scientific subjects ALEXANDER took a special interest in social problems. He was school medical officer for otology and was actively involved in the establishment of Austria's first kindergarten for deaf-mutes, which was established in 1916. Likewise, ALEXANDER helped to ease the lot of blind deaf-mutes, whose little institution in Vienna's district of Hietzing he supported.
ALEXANDER developed a number of new instruments, such as the ALEXANDER-syringe. He also modernized otological surgery by introducing a proper surgical team for otological operations. He himself paid for and established a modern histological laboratory which became the center for his and his students' research. His assistants were among others Oskar BENESI, Hans BRUNNER, Alexander CEMACH, Josef FISCHER, Rudolf LEIDLER, Josef SCHMIERER, Ignatz SOMMER, and Leopold STEIN.
ALEXANDER also collaborated with Robert BÁRÁNY (1876–1936; M.D. 1900, lecturer 1909, full professor [Uppsala] 1926), another student of POLITZER, on the chapter of Viennese research of the vestibular organ. In 1915 Robert BÁRÁNY was awarded the 1914 Nobel Prize for physiology and medicine "for his work on the physiology and pathology of the vestibular apparatus".[62] – Today BÁRÁNY's ways of investigation as well as his research concerning the function of the vestibular apparatus are of immense interest for aeronautics. His work is best summed up in his Nobel lecture, given on September 11, 1916:[63] ". . . As you will know, the inner

weiteren Arbeiten die Unerregbarkeit des Vestibularapparates bei Akustikustumoren und das nach ihm benannte Syndrom des Kleinhirnbrückenwinkels. Durch seine Untersuchungen wurde BÁRÁNY zum Begründer eines neuen Spezialgebietes der Ohrenheilkunde, der Oto-Neurologie, eines Grenzgebietes, das der bis dahin eng begrenzten Otologie eine ganz hervorragende Bedeutung und Stellung im Rahmen der Gesamtmedizin brachte.

BÁRÁNY beschäftigte sich auch mit ausgedehnten Untersuchungen über die Einwirkung des Alkohols bzw. der Alkoholvergiftung auf den Vestibularapparat. Einer der Studenten, die sich ihm für Versuche zur Verfügung stellten, war Franz FREMEL[65] (1887–1974; Dr. med. 1913, Dozent 1927, Vorstand der HNO-Ambulanz am Wilhelminenspital in Wien 1937, tit. a. o. Prof. 1941). Die Studenten wurden durch größere Alkoholmengen in schwere Rauschzustände versetzt und dann die Vestibularisprüfungen durchgeführt. So lernte FREMEL bereits als Student am eigenen Körper diese experimentellen Untersuchungsmethoden unter physiologischen und extrem pathologischen Bedingungen kennen; später beschäftigte er sich selbst intensiv mit diesen für die Oto-Neurologie so wichtigen Methoden. 1914 assistierte FREMEL auch bei den ersten in Wien von BÁRÁNY durchgeführten Fenestrationen bei Otosklerose, Operationen, die damals im Bereiche des hinteren Bogenganges möglichst weit weg vom Antrum wegen der Gefahr der Infektion durchgeführt wurden. Ebenfalls aus Sorge vor Komplikationen hatte URBANTSCHITSCH diese Operationen an seiner Klinik verboten, so daß BÁRÁNY mit FREMEL als Assistenten in einer Privatklinik operieren mußte.

BÁRÁNYS Einstellung zur Wissenschaft ist vielleicht am besten durch die Worte charakterisiert, die er bei einer Dankesadresse für eine wissenschaftliche Auszeichnung sprach: „Die Tätigkeit des Forschers gliedert sich in drei Unterabteilungen: Erstens, er muß scharf beobachten, Wichtiges von Unwichtigem sondern, muß selbständig denken, selbständig die Schlüsse aus dem Gefundenen ziehen. ... In zweiter Linie muß der Forscher aber, wenn er etwas gefunden hat, mit aller Energie dafür eintreten und dafür kämpfen. Zu oft sehe ich beim Studium der Literatur, wie ganz wichtige Tatsachen ganz einfach dadurch, daß ihr Entdecker sich nicht genügend dafür einsetzte, wieder untergehen und vergessen werden. Die dritte Tätigkeit, die der Forscher entfalten muß, soll er das Maximum der Energien entwickeln, die er zu entwickeln fähig ist, besteht in der Organisation wissenschaftlicher Arbeit in der Gründung einer Schule. Denn der einzelne für sich allein ist ja im Laufe eines kurzen Lebens doch nur imstande, einen kleinen Bruchteil der Fragen zu bearbeiten und zu lösen, die sich ihm darbieten."[66]

Nach Emil SCHLANDER lieferten BÁRÁNYS Forschungsergebnisse für den Neurologen wichtige Anhaltspunkte in der Krankheitserkenntnis und Lokalisation im Bereiche des zentralen Vestibularis, im Verlauf seiner Verbindungen mit den Augenmuskelkernen, dem Kleinhirn und Rückenmark. Die zunehmenden Erfahrungen auf diesem Gebiet bereicherten in gleicher Weise die Neurologie, die Ophthalmologie und die Otologie. Durch die bedeutenden Fortschritte in der Diagnostik der Labyrintherkrankungen wurde nunmehr eine systematische chirurgische Therapie dieser Erkrankungen in die Wege geleitet. „Mit BÁRÁNY und NEUMANN hatte ALEXANDER ... wesentlichen Anteil am Ausbau der ... Erforschung der Labyrintherkrankungen und deren Komplikationen. Die

ear, not only in humans but also in all vertebrates, consists of the cochlea for the purpose of hearing and the vestibulo-semicircular canals. ... Up until the 19th century there was a complete lack of knowledge of its function. The first to begin experimental investigations in this field was the celebrated French physiologist FLOURENS. His investigations were published in 1825. FLOURENS thought that it would be possible to get an insight into the function of the semi-circular canal apparatus by destroying it. In fact, these experiments which were undertaken with pigeons, rabbits and other animals produced quite remarkable, constant and previously unknown disturbances. For instance, if the horizontal semi-circular canal was destroyed in a pigeon, it went on turning horizontally in a circle. If a vertical semi-circular canal was destroyed, the pigeon turned somersaults. FLOURENS has described the phenomena extremely well. But he did not give an explanation. In particular, he did not have the faintest idea that the animals were suffering from vertigo. ... Also, the work of a great physiologist in Prague, PURKINJE, was unknown to FLOURENS, although PURKINJE was actually, in the same year, investigating the phenomena of vertigo in humans. PURKINJE tried out his experiments partly on himself and partly on mentally sick persons, ... PURKINJE has discovered the involuntary movements of the eyeball during vertigo, the nystagmus of the eyes, about which we shall be speaking a great deal ... He knew of FLOURENS' work. But strangely enough he too did not realize that FLOURENS' animals were suffering from vertigo, nor that in the spot where certain sensations arise there must be a sensory organ present which receives them. ... As neither of these two great research scientists was able to find the solution to the mystery, it is small wonder that none of their contemporaries were able to do so either. ... Only in the year 1861 was a Frenchman, MÉNIÈRE, able to take a bold step forward. ... He was an otologist and had observed from a purely clinical standpoint the frequent coincidence of vertigo, 'Schwerhörigkeit' and tinnitus in cases with normal middle ear. The site of hearing was now known to be in the cochlea. Its destruction or impairment causes the tinnitus and the 'Schwerhörigkeit'. Vertigo, it was thought at the time, could only be caused by a disease of the cerebellum. He observed this kind of patient for years and saw absolutely no symptoms of brain disease. ... MÉNIÈRE now had the idea that the vertigo phenomena were symptoms of disease in the semi-circular canal apparatus and he now succeeded, where FLOURENS and PURKINJE had failed, in seeing through the confusing diversity of the vertigo manifestations in humans and in animals and recognizing that those animals whose semi-circular canals had been operated upon by FLOURENS had vertigo ... In 1874, three men arrived all at the same time at a theory concerning the semi-circular canal apparatus which is even today, broadly speaking, correct. These were a general practitioner ... Dr. Josef BREUER in Vienna, the Viennese physicist and philosopher, Ernst MACH, and the American, CRUM BROWN, in Philadelphia. ... BREUER started by repeating FLOURENS's experiments with pigeons with improved technique and came directly to the conviction that movement of the fluid in the semi-circular canals, the endolymph, gave rise to the FLOURENS phenomena. ... MACH ... first established the mathematical equations for rotary movements. Then he made some investigations with human subjects to ascertain whether there was any evidence of a sensory organ

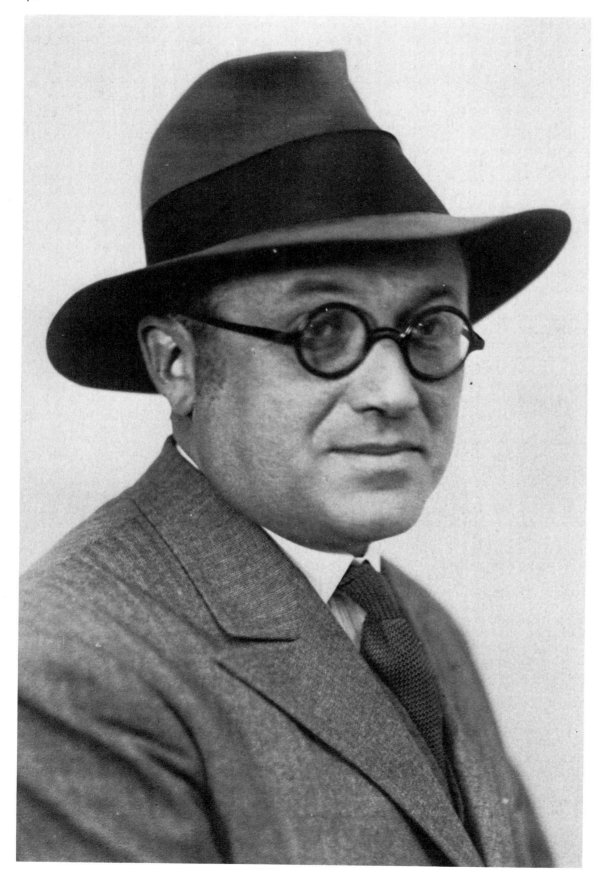

Hans Brunner

Wiener Schule, mit den Genannten an der Spitze, eroberte sich mit diesen medizinischen Großtaten neuerlich die führende Stellung in der otologischen Wissenschaft. ALEXANDER, BÁRÁNY und NEUMANN schufen neue Grundlagen der modernen Labyrinthforschung, die der Ohrenheilkunde einen ungeahnten Aufschwung brachte. In der Verleihung des Nobelpreises an BÁRÁNY fand dessen wissenschaftliche Arbeit die internationale Anerkennung."[67]

Am 12. April 1932 kam Gustav ALEXANDER im 58. Lebensjahr unter tragischen Umständen ums Leben: ALEXANDER hatte 1905 noch unter POLITZER bei einem Patienten mit einer Sattelnase eine Nasenplastik durchgeführt. Der Patient, mit dem Operationsresultat unzufrieden, klagte auf Schadenersatz. Nach Abweisung der Klage wurde der Patient vom Chirurgen O. FÖDERL operiert. Nach neuerlicher Klage gegen FÖDERL, dann gegen ALEXANDER, schoß 1910 der Patient auf ALEXANDER, der dem Anschlag entging. Der Patient wurde für geisteskrank erklärt, der Heilanstalt Steinhof übergeben und 1922 aus Österreich abgeschoben. 1932 kehrte der Patient nach Wien zurück und erschoß ALEXANDER.

Zum Nachfolger ALEXANDERS an der Poliklinik wurde Hans BRUNNER (1893–1955) ernannt, der seit 1921 Assistent bei ALEXANDER gewesen war und 1932 habilitiert wurde. Wie sein Lehrer ALEXANDER beschäftigte sich auch BRUNNER mit Vorliebe mit der Histo-Pathologie des Schläfenbeines. In zahlreichen Arbeiten hat er seine Untersuchungen über die otologische Hirndiagnostik, die er in jahrelanger Arbeit an dem reichen Tumormaterial der Wiener Nervenklinik angestellt hatte, niedergelegt, als deren Ergebnis 1936 seine Monographie „Otologische Diagnostik der Hirntumoren" erschien. Für das von ihm redigierte Handbuch der Neurologie des Ohres schrieb er eine Reihe wertvoller Beiträge. Operativ hat BRUNNER im Sinne ALEXANDERS weitergearbeitet, sich u. a. mit der Ausarbeitung plastischer Operationen bei Fazialislähmung beschäftigt. Unter BRUNNER stieg die Ambulanzfrequenz auf 6.000 neue Patienten im Jahr an. 1938 mußte BRUNNER seine langjährige Arbeitsstätte verlassen und fand in den Vereinigten Staaten eine neue Heimat mit reicher Arbeitsmöglichkeit, zuerst in Chicago, bei Fr. LEDERER, dann in Newark, wo er 1955 starb.

Nach BRUNNER übernahm Hermann MARSCHIK (1878–1969), der seit 1920 die Abteilung für Hals- und Nasenkrankheiten geführt hatte, auch die Ohrenabteilung der Poliklinik und vereinigte somit erstmalig seit der Gründung der Anstalt beide Fachabteilungen. Auf MARSCHIK wird im folgenden Abschnitt noch zurückzukommen sein. Ihm folgte im Dezember 1946 als Vorstand der HNO-Abteilung der Allgemeinen Poliklinik Eduard Herbert MAJER (geb. 1909), die er bis 1976 führte. Sein Nachfolger wurde E. MORITSCH (geb. 1926).

Heinrich NEUMANN (1873–1939; Dr. med. 1898, Doz. 1907, Tit. a. o. Prof. 1911, a. o. Prof. 1919), der POLITZER-Schüler, dessen Tradition er fortsetzte, übernahm 1919 die Leitung der Wiener Ohrenklinik. In seinem Referat über die konservative Radikaloperation trat er bereits 1928 ganz im heutigen Sinne für ein schonendes, die Funktion erhaltendes Vorgehen ein. Auf den atypischen Verlauf der Mukosusotitis, die oft nach einer wochenlangen Latenzzeit zur Mastoiditis und tödlichen Komplikationen führte, hat NEUMANN immer wieder hingewiesen. Bei der Mastoiditis trat er für die komplette Mastoidektomie, die systematische Zellausräumung, ein, da früher

capable of perceiving rotary motion. . . . CRUM BROWN solved the problem in yet another way. He investigated a number of persons with regard to their vertigo symptoms and without much further thought he came directly to the assumption that the semi-circular canal mechanism must be the sensory organ capable of apprehending these quite specific sensations. . . . In spite of the pioneer work of all these men, however, the whole field of diseases of the semi-circular canals in humans was veiled in obscurity. It was impossible to understand all the phenomena observed, for there was no real method for testing the function of the apparatus such as had long since been carried out for other sensory organs." At this point BÁRÁNY's research set in: "As a young otologist I worked in Professor POLITZER's Clinic in Vienna. Among my patients there were many who required syringing of the ears. A number of them complained afterwards of vertigo. Obviously I examined their eyes and I noticed in doing this that there was a nystagmus in a certain direction. I made a note of this. After a time, when I had collected about twenty of these observations, I compared them one with another and was amazed always to find the same note. I then realized that some general principle must be implied, but at the time I did not understand it. Chance came to my aid. One of my patients, whose ears I was syringing, said to me: 'Doctor, I only get giddy when the water is not warm enough. When I do my own ears at home and use warm enough water I never get giddy.' I then called the nurse and asked her to get me warmer water for the syringe. She maintained that it was already warm enough. I replied that if the patient found it too cold we should conform to his wish. The next time she brought me very hot water in the bowl. When I syringed the patient's ear he shouted: 'But Doctor, this water is much too hot and now I am giddy again.' I quickly observed his eyes and noticed that the nystagmus was in an exactly opposite direction from the previous one when cold water had been used."[64] – The explanation was now clear. The decisive factor was the temperature of the syringing fluid and it was soon also clear that the phenomenon, the so-called *caloric reaction*, proceeded from the semi-circular canals, in which the endolymph increases in specific gravity with cooling, showing a tendency to sink, whereas with warming the specific gravity decreases and the fluid shows a tendency to rise. The caloric reaction for the first time provided otology with a method of investigation of the excitability of the vestibular apparatus which can be used in practically all cases. If the reaction is positive, then the canals are excitable, i.e., not totally destroyed; if it is negative then they are destroyed – with a few, easily checked exceptions. This very simply obtained reaction has become basic for the understanding of, and therefore for the therapeutic handling of, a number of labyrinth diseases – in particular those of an inflammatory nature. BÁRÁNY also studied systematically the other vestibular reactions. He provided an explanation for the vestibular phenomena occurring after rotation which was in sharp contrast to what had been thought before and established the clinical and physiological importance of the so-called rotatory reaction. He also studied the remaining phenomena of the vestibular syndrome, both the subjective and the objective ones, and systematized them. Here he was chiefly concerned with developing the question of the so-called vestibular reaction movements. First of all he established that vestibular disturbances of equilibrium, which were already known, occur in a

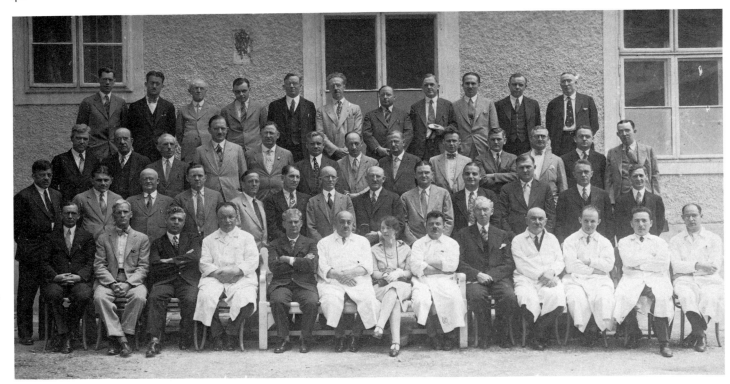

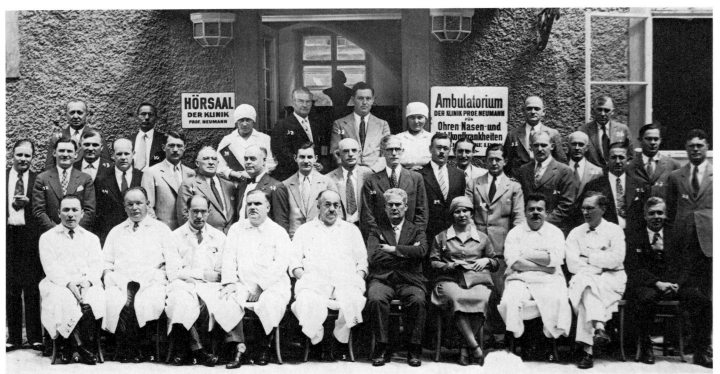

Oben und unten: Heinrich Neumann, Bildmitte, sitzend, mit Teilnehmern an sogenannten „Amerikaner-Kursen". Mackenzie-Group der Jahre 1929 und 1930. Auf dem unteren Bild u. a. links von Neumann, sitzend: Schlander, Eisinger, Buchband und Tamari. Rechts von Neumann: Mackenzie.

Top and bottom: Heinrich Neumann, seated in the middle of the first row, with participants of the so-called "Courses for Americans." The Mackenzie group of the years 1929 and 1930. In the bottom picture to the left of Neumann among others: Schlander, Eisinger, Buchband and Tamari, all seated. To the right of Neumann: Mackenzie.

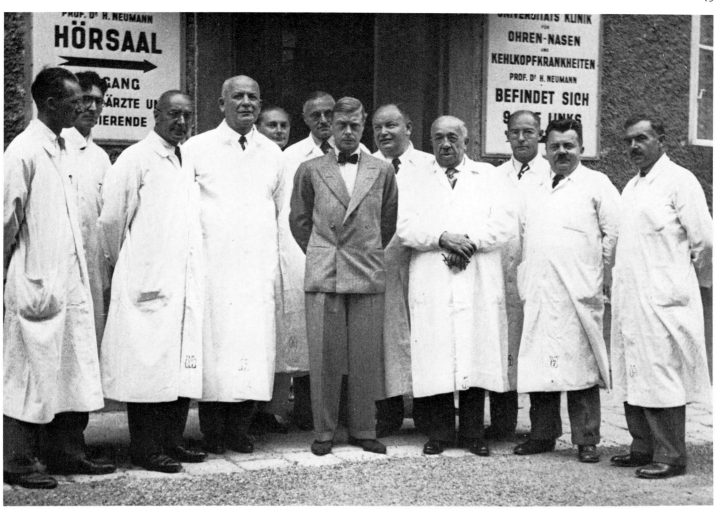

Heinrich Neumann, Vorstand der Universitäts-Klinik für Ohren-, Nasen- und Kehlkopfkrankheiten, behandelte im Jahr 1936 den englischen König Edward VIII.
Neben dem König von England und Neumann sind folgende Klinikassistenten zu sehen (von links nach rechts): Majer, Bauer, Popper, Hofrat Glaser, Jents, Wiethe, Buchband, Eisinger, Fremel, Wessely.

Heinrich Neumann, head of the University Clinic of Ear, Nose and Throat Diseases, treated the English King Edward VIII in 1936.
Next to the King of England and Neumann are the following assistants (from left to right): Majer, Bauer, Popper, Hofrat Glaser, Jents, Wiethe, Buchband, Eisinger, Fremel, Wessely.

häufig von zurückgelassenen Zellen Komplikationen ausgingen. Bei der otogenen Meningitis hat er die sog. Meningitisoperation angegeben. Mit gewissem Stolz konnte NEUMANN 1926 in seinem Überblick über die „Entwicklungsphasen und Leistungen der Ohrenheilkunde" in der ‚Wiener klinischen Wochenschrift' feststellen: „Wenn wir das vergangene Vierteljahrhundert überblicken, so können wir uns ruhig sagen, dass wir trotz der Unterbrechung durch die Kriegswirren gute Arbeit geleistet haben, was insoferne von der übrigen Medizin anerkannt wurde, als sich doch die Einsicht durchgerungen hat, dass die Ohrenheilkunde mit ihren innigen Zusammenhängen mit anderen grossen Gebieten, mit ihrer Fülle von lebensbedrohenden Krankheitsbildern, unbedingt zum Rüstzeug des praktizierenden Arztes gehört und als ein den anderen Disziplinen ebenbürtiges Fach unter die Prüfungsfächer aufgenommen wurde. Das erste Viertel unseres Jahrhunderts ist beendet, wir haben es wie im Fluge durchlebt und stehen jetzt an der Wende zum zweiten Viertel und schon drängen sich die Fragen nach der Lösung von Problemen, deren auch die Ohrenheilkunde eine stattliche Reihe hat. Nicht im Rahmen des Spezialgebietes sind sie unserer Meinung nach zu lösen, sondern im lebendigen Kontakt mit der Gesamtmedizin und ihren Hilfswissenschaften. Von dem Ausbau der Serologie, der Lehre der endokrinen Drüsen usw., erwarten wir den Anstoss, der uns im zweiten Viertel des Jahrhunderts einen Schritt vorwärts bringen wird, ungestört durch äussere Ereignisse, so hoffen und wünschen wir es!"[68]

NEUMANN hatte eine große internationale Praxis, hatte, wie es heißt, „das Ohr der Könige", behandelte den spanischen und rumänischen König, 1936 den englischen König.

Knapp vor dem Einmarsch der deutschen Truppen in Wien hielt NEUMANN am 11. März 1938 seine letzte Vorlesung und wurde kurz darauf verhaftet, jedoch nach einigen Tagen auf Intervention des Herzogs VON WINDSOR wieder freigelassen. In den nächsten Monaten führte NEUMANN zahlreiche Auslandsreisen mit Genehmigung der deutschen Regierung durch, um Geld für die jüdische Emigration aufzutreiben, so auch im Juli 1938 zu der von ROOSEVELT einberufenen ersten Flüchtlingskonferenz in Evian. Der Schriftsteller Hans HABE hat seinen Roman „Die Mission" dem Andenken NEUMANNS gewidmet und dessen Aufgabe in Evian unter einem Pseudonym für NEUMANN geschildert. Am 5. November 1939 ist NEUMANN an den Folgen eines Leberkarzinoms in New York gestorben. Leopold ARZT fand 1946 ergreifende Worte für seinen Freund NEUMANN. Die realistische Schilderung der Situation in NEUMANNS Wartezimmer spricht nicht nur für den Weltruf des Otologen, sondern auch dafür, daß NEUMANN einer von den vielen Ärzten war, die Kaiser Josephs II. Widmungswunsch für das Allgemeine Krankenhaus, „saluti et solatio aegrorum", also „Zum Wohl und zum Trost der Kranken", wirklich realisieren konnten: „NEUMANN war einer jener wenigen Männer, in dessen Ordination sich die Kranken aller Stände und aller Nationen einfanden. Neben dem gekrönten Herrscher saß der Präsident einer Republik, neben seinen ärmsten flüchtigen Glaubensgenossen aus dem Osten waren höchste kirchliche Würdenträger, indische Maharadschas und Hocharistokraten anzutreffen. Unterschiede durch Geburt und Abstammung, durch Nation, Konfession und soziale Stellung waren verschwunden. Er war der Arzt für alle Kranken, die seine Hilfe suchten, und ihre Zahl war groß."[69]

In GRAZ[70] lasen die Privatdozenten Johannes KESSEL regular manner, in a certain relationship to the existing nystagmus, so that change of position, or tendency to change of position, always occurs in the same plane but in an opposite direction to the existing nystagmus. From this follows the interesting and clinically extraordinarily important fact that existing vestibular imbalance changes direction with an alteration in the head position. These imbalances, which may stem from the muscular apparatus of the trunk, correspond with other analogous phenomena in all the other muscles which are directed by the will. With an appropriate series of experiments it can be shown how each extremity, or part of an extremity, deviates from a certain position, or tends to deviate, in the same plane but in an opposite direction to the nystagmus caused, or already present. This previously quite unknown phenomenon has become, through BÁRÁNY's so-called pointing test, an integral part of the examination methods of otologists and neurologists.

BÁRÁNY also studied the influence of alcohol and alcoholic poisoning on the vestibular apparatus of human beings. One of the students who placed himself at BÁRÁNY's disposal for the tests was Franz FREMEL[65] (1887–1974; M.D. 1913, lecturer 1927, head of the ENT-out-patient department of the Wilhelminen Hospital in Vienna in 1937, "titular" associate professor 1941). Later FREMEL himself carried out scientific work in this field. In 1914 he also assisted BÁRÁNY when he carried out his fenestrations caused by otosclerosis. These were the first operations of this kind in Vienna. URBANTSCHITSCH had forbidden these operations at his clinic because he was afraid of complications. Therefore, BÁRÁNY with FREMEL assisting had to use a private clinic.

BÁRÁNY's involvement with science was best summed up by himself: "The work of a researcher can be divided into three categories: first, he needs a sharp and clear perception, must be able to separate the important facts from the less important ones, and must also be able to think independently. Secondly, the researcher must defend his results with all his energy; he must even fight for them. I very often find that important facts are being neglected and even forgotten only because their discoverer did not stand up for them sufficiently. Lastly, the researcher must invest the maximum of his energies into founding his own school of followers, for a single person can only – in his short life span – deal with and solve a fraction of the questions that need to be solved."[66]

According to Emil SCHLANDER, BÁRÁNY's research provided the neurologist with important clues in the diagnosis of diseases of the central vestibular apparatus, in its connection with the nucleus of the ocular muscles, the cerebellum and the spinal cord, and he continued: "BÁRÁNY, NEUMANN, and ALEXANDER are the ones who have to be credited for the research and development concerning the treatment of diseases of the labyrinth. The Vienna School, headed by these three men, again took the leading position in otology and BÁRÁNY's work found its international recognition by the Nobel Prize which he was awarded."[67]

On April 12, 1932, Gustav ALEXANDER's life came to a dramatic end: in 1905, still working under POLITZER, ALEXANDER had performed a saddle nose operation. The patient, dissatisfied with the operation, sued for damages, however, unsuccessfully. Later the surgeon O. FÖDERL performed a reconstructive operation. The patient, still dissatisfied, now sued both ALEXANDER and FÖDERL but again was denied compensation. As a result of this law-suit the patient tried to

(1839–1907) – von 1875 bis zu seiner Berufung nach Jena 1886 – und Karl EMELE über Ohrenheilkunde. Da es eine Klinik für das Spezialfach noch nicht gab, mußten die Vorlesungen und Krankenvorstellungen im Hörsaal der Augenklinik stattfinden. Der POLITZER-Schüler KESSEL durchtrennte im Dezember 1875 bei einer Patientin mit großer Trommelfellperforation, fehlendem Hammer und Amboß, narbiger Fixation des Stapes, hochgradiger Schwerhörigkeit und quälenden Ohrgeräuschen die Narben um den Steigbügel, wodurch es zu einer Hörverbesserung und Verschwinden der Ohrgeräusche kam. Dies war die erste Steigbügelmobilisation; die erste Stapesextraktion zur Hörverbesserung führte KESSEL 1878 durch. 1879 beschrieb er Hörverbesserungen durch Abdeckung des runden Fensters, weiters Hörerfolge durch Fixation des Trommelfells an das Stapesköpfchen. Durch diese Eingriffe wurde KESSEL zum Begründer der hörverbessernden Chirurgie. 1886 folgte KESSEL einem Ruf als Professor der Ohrenheilkunde an die Universität Jena.

Damit trat in Graz eine Pause ein, während der die Ohrenkrankheiten (und auch die Hals- und Nasenkrankheiten) im Rahmen der inneren Medizin Vertretung fanden. 1890 wurde Johann HABERMANN (1849–1935; Dr. med. 1875), 1886 in Prag als Privatdozent für Ohrenheilkunde habilitiert, als Extraordinarius der Ohrenheilkunde nach Graz berufen. Nach großen anfänglichen Schwierigkeiten wurden ihm im alten Paulustorspital drei Räume zur Verfügung gestellt, die als Operationssaal, Ambulanz und Hörsaal dienen mußten; dazu gab es einige Not-Gastbetten in der chirurgischen Abteilung. Zwei angrenzende Zimmer mit sechs Betten für Männer und drei für Frauen kamen dann dazu und so konnte am 1. Oktober 1893 die Klinik für Ohren-, Nasen- und Halskranke an der Universität Graz eröffnet werden. Nur langsam wurden HABERMANN Erweiterungen möglich gemacht, bis er 1913 die neue Klinik in Graz mit sechzig Betten und allen erforderlichen Nebenräumen beziehen konnte. An Ärzten standen ihm anfangs ein Assistent und ein Sekundararzt zur Verfügung, ab 1903 noch ein zweiter Assistent.

HABERMANN wurde 1899 Titular-, 1913 wirklicher Ordinarius. Von ihm stammt eine der ersten Arbeiten über berufsbedingte Schwerhörigkeit bei einem Kesselschmied. „Es ist zweifellos eine prophetische Tat HABERMANNS, daß er für das Ohr anatomisch nachwies, wie schädlich sich Lärm auswirken kann. Seit damals hat man die Schädigung auch anderer Organe durch Lärm als Tatsache festgestellt", schreibt MESSERKLINGER.[71] In weiteren Untersuchungen konnte HABERMANN die Cholesteatomentstehung durch Einwanderung der Epidermis in das Mittelohr feststellen.[72]

HABERMANN hielt von Anfang an auch Vorlesungen über Nase und Rachen, während die Laryngologie noch bei den Internisten verblieb. Im Wintersemester 1895/96 las HABERMANN neben der „Klinik der Krankheiten des Ohres" eine besondere „Klinik der Krankheiten der Nase und des Halses", eine Lehrveranstaltung, die er im Sommersemester 1896 „Klinik der Nasen-, Rachen- und Kehlkopfkrankheiten" nannte, d. h. man verzichtete „auf getrennte Lehrstühle und Kliniken".[73]

Unter HABERMANNS Schülern finden wir eine Reihe hervorragender Otologen, wie Otto BARNICK, Karl BAUERREISS, Karl BIEHL, Max KRASSNIG, Otto MAYER, Erich PHLEPS und Walter STUPKA.

Nach der Emeritierung HABERMANNS wegen Erreichung der Altersgrenze im Jahr 1922 wurde Johannes ZANGE

shoot ALEXANDER but failed. The patient was admitted to a psychiatric clinic and later left Austria. In 1932 he returned to Austria and shot ALEXANDER.

ALEXANDER was succeeded by Hans BRUNNER (1893–1955) at the Policlinic. BRUNNER, an assistant of ALEXANDER since 1921 and lecturer since 1932, concerned himself primarily with the histo-pathology of the temporal bone. He also published several scientific papers on otological brain diagnosis from the great number of tumor patients he had treated at the Viennese mental hospital. In 1936 his monograph "Otological Diagnosis of Brain Tumors" appeared. BRUNNER continued the surgical work which ALEXANDER had initiated, and also devoted himself to the technique of plastic surgery in cases of facial paralysis. During BRUNNER's time the outpatient department at the Policlinic was frequented by 6,000 patients every year. BRUNNER had to leave Austria in 1938. He emigrated to the United States where he found a new home, working at first in Chicago and then in Newark, where he died in 1955.

Hermann MARSCHIK (1878–1969), who since 1920 had headed the department of nose- and throat-diseases, took over BRUNNER's otological department at the Policlinic. Now for the first time in the history of the Policlinic both departments were united. (We will refer to MARSCHIK in more detail in the second part of our book.) In December 1946, Eduard Herbert MAJER (born in 1909) was appointed head of the department, which he directed until 1976. He was succeeded by E. MORITSCH (born in 1926).

In 1919 Heinrich NEUMANN (1873–1939; M. D. 1898, lecturer 1907, "titular" associate professor 1911, associate professor 1919), another student of POLITZER, whose tradition he continued, became head of the University Clinic of Otology. His main work was in intracranial complications of purulent inflammation of the middle ear. In 1928 he gave a lecture on conservative radical operations and he advocated a function preserving surgical technique. He also pointed to the atypical course of mucosus otitis, which very often – after a latent period of several weeks – led to life-threatening complications. In regard to mastoiditis NEUMANN was for complete mastoidectomy and systematic cell removal. He was also a pioneer of the surgical treatment of meningitis. He proudly stated in his survey entitled "Phases of Development and Achievements in Otology" in 1926: "Looking back at the past quarter of a century we may say that despite the interruption caused by World War One we have been able to achieve good and solid work in our specialty; work which has been recognized by the representatives of the other branches of medicine. It has become common belief that otology with its close connections with other branches of medicine, with its great number of life-threatening aspects has to be included into the medical curriculum. We have now completed the first quarter of the new century and new problems have to be solved. In my opinion they can only be solved if otology is practiced and taught in close connection with all other fields of medicine. The expansion of serology, the science of the ductless glands, etc. shall bring the new impetus that will enable us to cope with the demands of the second quarter of the new century, hopefully undisturbed by outward influences."[68]

NEUMANN had a large international clientele; he had "the ear of Kings", since among his patients were the King of Spain, of Rumania, and in 1936 the King of England.

Shortly before the occupation of Austria by German troops in

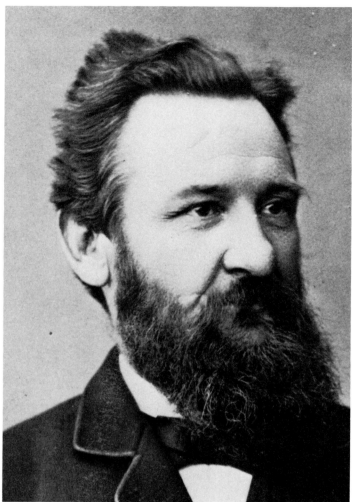

Johannes Kessel führte 1875 in Graz die erste Stapesmobilisation durch.

In 1875 Kessel, a former student of Politzer's, performed the first stapes mobilization.

(1880–1969; Dr. med. 1907 [Halle], Dozent 1913 [Jena], a. o. Prof. 1919 [Jena]) an die Universität Graz berufen. Damals lag bereits eine Periode fruchtbarsten wissenschaftlichen Schaffens hinter ihm. 1919 war seine Monographie über die „Pathologische Anatomie und Physiologie der mittelohrentspringenden Labyrinthentzündungen" erschienen als Ergebnis einer jahrelangen, mit größter Konsequenz betriebenen Forschung. Schon während seiner Ausbildung in pathologischer Anatomie bei Eugen FRAENKEL in Hamburg richtete ZANGE sein Augenmerk auf die Veränderungen am menschlichen Ohrlabyrinth. In den folgenden Jahren als Assistent und Oberarzt bei MANASSE in Straßburg und bei WITTMAACK in Jena bearbeitete er unter Zugrundelegung des großen pathohistologischen Materials die Labyrinthentzündungen und habilitierte sich auf diesem Gebiet in Jena. Als das oben genannte Werk in seiner endgültigen Fassung vorlag, „waren damit die Richtlinien für die konservative und operative Behandlung der Labyrinthentzündungen und ihrer Folgeerkrankungen im Schädel gegeben"[74]. Die ersten Jahre von ZANGES Grazer Tätigkeit waren der oto- und rhinogenen Meningitis einschließlich der traumatischen Meningitis gewidmet. Von ZANGE und KINDLER wurde der Zysternenblock bei raumbeengenden Prozessen im Schädel beschrieben. Unter ZANGE wurde die Grazer Klinik wesentlich erweitert und ausgebaut.

1938 NEUMANN held his last lecture on March 11, 1938. Shortly afterward he was arrested, but was soon set free due to the intervention of the Duke of Windsor. During the following months he frequently travelled abroad to raise money for the emigration of his fellow Jews. In July 1938 he was summoned to the Refugee Conference in Evian which President ROOSEVELT had called for. The author Hans HABE made NEUMANN the main character of his novel "The Mission" which is based on this episode.

On November 5, 1939, NEUMANN died in New York. In 1946 his colleague Leopold ARZT found moving words for his friend NEUMANN. The realistic description of the milieu of NEUMANN's waiting room given by ARZT not only accounts for the international reputation of NEUMANN but is also a true example of a physician living according to the motto inscribed above the entrance of the Vienna General Hospital *"Saluti et Solatio Aegrorum"*. According to ARZT, "NEUMANN was one of the few physicians whose waiting room was filled with patients stemming from all classes and nations. Next to the crowned sovereign sat the president of a republic; next to the poorest fugitive fellow-believer from the East sat a high dignitary of the church and next to him maybe a maharajah from India or a high ranking aristocrat. In NEUMANN's waiting room there existed no difference of birth, descent, nation-

Johann Habermann

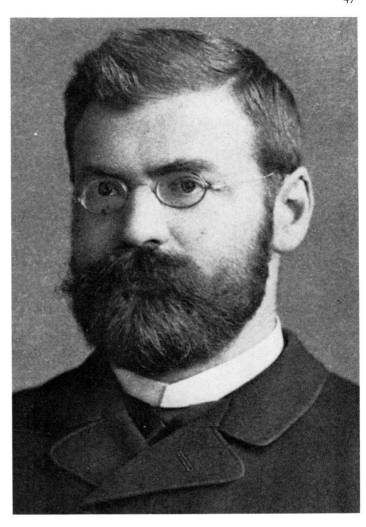

Auf eine Anregung von Gustav HOFER (1887–1970), der nach der Berufung von ZANGE nach Jena 1931 die Grazer Klinik übernommen hatte, wurde von F. X. KOCH der günstige Einfluß männlicher Sexualhormone auf die Altersschwerhörigkeit nachgewiesen. Über HOFER schreibt sein Nachfolger an der Grazer Klinik (1959), Walter MESSERKLINGER (geb. 1920): „1913 kam er als Operateur an die Klinik EISELSBERG, nahm am Ersten Weltkrieg zuerst als Arzt eines Fronttruppenteils teil, wurde dann in die Chirugentruppe v. EISELSBERG versetzt und übernahm schließlich die Führung einer großen Verwundetenabteilung. Anschließend übersiedelte er als Assistent an die Laryngo-Rhinologische Klinik Ottokar v. CHIARIS; Markus HAJEK [CHIARIS Nachfolger] übernahm ihn als Ersten Assistenten. Hier wirkte HOFER in führender Stellung an der Entwicklung unseres Faches mit: Durch Einführung einer Reihe namhafter Verbesserungen wurde in jener Zeit die große Larynxchirurgie weiter ausgebaut; aus aller Welt kamen viele Fachkollegen nach Wien als einem Zentrum der Laryngologie und wurden in Spezialvorlesungen und Kursen weitergeschult, und schließlich entstand damals durch Vereinigung der Rhino-Laryngologie mit der Otologie unsere heutige Spezialdisziplin, die Hals-Nasen-Ohren-Heilkunde. 1931 folgte Prof. HOFER einem Ruf der Universität Graz, um nach KESSEL, HABERMANN und ZANGE die große

ality, confession, or color. He was the physician for all patients who sought his help, and their number was large."[69]
In GRAZ[70] lectures in otology were given by the private lecturers Johannes KESSEL (1839–1907) and Karl EMELE. Since a department for the specialty had not yet been founded, both lectures and demonstrations had to take place in the lecture theatre of the ophthalmological clinic.
In December 1875, KESSEL, a former student of POLITZER, performed the first stapes mobilization. In 1878 he also performed the first stapes extraction, and in 1879 he described methods to improve hearing by covering the round fenestra and by fixation of the tympanic membrane to the head of the stapes. KESSEL thus became the father of the surgical improvement of hearing. In 1886 KESSEL received a call to Jena to become professor of otology there. When he left, otology as well as laryngology and rhinology were no longer represented in Graz, but were dealt with as part of internal medicine.
In 1890 Johann HABERMANN (1849–1935; M. D. 1875), who in 1886 had become private lecturer of otology in Prague, was called to Graz. He had to face a great number of difficulties, but was finally assigned three rooms at the old Paulustor-Hospital. These rooms served as operating rooms, out-patient department and lecture rooms. For his surgical cases two beds were reserved at the surgical clinic. Later two adjacent rooms

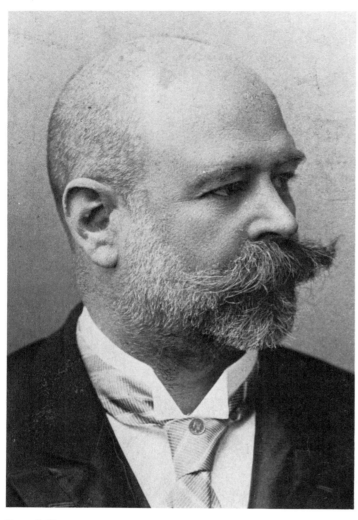

Georg Juffinger

Tradition dieser Lehrkanzel bis zu seiner Emeritierung 1959 fortzuführen. . . . Seine ganz hervorragende Schaffenskraft galt der Grundlagenforschung in der Rhino-Laryngologie und der Verschmelzung der Otologie mit der Nasen- und Kehlkopfheilkunde zu einer unzertrennlichen Einheit."[75]
Im INNSBRUCKER Vorlesungsverzeichnis finden sich für die Jahre von 1869 bis 1891 keine Ankündigungen über Vorlesungen aus dem Gebiet der Ohrenheilkunde wie auch der Laryngologie, so daß man wohl mit Recht annehmen darf, daß etwaiger Unterricht ohne ausdrückliche Erwähnung von Internisten oder Chirurgen erteilt wurde. 1893 wurde Georg JUFFINGER (1853–1913) zum Extraordinarius für Rhinologie, Laryngologie und Otiatrie ernannt und 1894 die Universitäts-Ohrenklinik in Innsbruck eröffnet. Die Ohrenklinik verfügte über sechs Betten (bei einem Belegraum von 662 m²) und es mag für JUFFINGER schwer genug gewesen sein, unter den beengten Verhältnissen den „Betrieb" dort einzurichten. Dies berichtet Ludwig HÖRBST (1903–1981) in der hervorragenden „Erinnerungsschrift der Universitätsklinik für Ohren-, Nasen- und Halskrankheiten in Innsbruck",[76] der wir nun auszugsweise folgen.
Der aus Hötting bei Innsbruck gebürtige JUFFINGER wurde 1881 in Innsbruck promoviert und habilitierte sich 1892 für Laryngologie in Wien. Bis zu seiner Berufung nach Innsbruck arbeitete er als Assistent bei SCHRÖTTER und dessen Nachfolger STOERK. Vom Ausbildungsgang her war JUFFINGER somit Laryngologe, versäumte es jedoch nie, auch in der Ohrenheilkunde reiche Erfahrung zu sammeln. Sein erfolgreichstes wissenschaftliches Arbeitsgebiet war das Sklerom und die Tuberkulose der Schleimhaut der oberen Luftwege. 1911 wurde JUFFINGER Ordinarius und leitete die Klinik bis zu seinem Tode im Jahre 1914.
Nach einer zweijährigen, durch den Ersten Weltkrieg bedingten Übergangszeit, in der die Klinik durch den Assistenten Karl GUGLER betreut wurde, erfolgte 1916 die Berufung von Heinrich HERZOG (1875–1938) zum Vorstand.
HERZOG, 1875 in Pfaffenburg (Bayern) geboren, studierte Medizin in München und Würzburg und wurde 1900 promoviert. HERZOG, der 1915 den Titel eines außerordentlichen Professors erhalten hatte, wurde aus seiner Felddienstleitung nach Innsbruck geholt. Er hatte von jeher eine besondere Vorliebe für experimentelle Arbeiten und machte sich durch seine Untersuchungen über die experimentelle Labyrinthitis einen besonderen Namen. Neben seiner wissenschaftlichen Tätigkeit widmete er sich ganz dem klinischen Betrieb, den er trotz der kriegs- und nachkriegsbedingten Schwierigkeiten wesentlich verbesserte. Es gelang ihm sogar, die Räumlichkeiten der Klinik zu erweitern und die Bettenzahl auf 26 zu erhöhen. Die überaus beengte Situation an der Klinik, die zu ändern es ihm nicht gelang, veranlaßten HERZOG, 1928 einen Ruf an die Universität München anzunehmen.
Nach dem Abgang Herzogs übernahm Wilfried KRAINZ (1895–1943) zunächst vertretungsweise die Ohren-, Nasen-, Halsklinik und wurde 1931 als a. o. Professor zum Vorstand ernannt; 1941 erfolgte seine Ernennung zum ordentlichen Professor. KRAINZ entfaltete eine sehr intensive wissenschaftliche Tätigkeit und publizierte zahlreiche Arbeiten über die Pneumatisation und die entzündlichen Erkrankungen des Warzenfortsatzes. Zahlreiche tierexperimentelle und histologische Studien über die Veränderungen der Labyrinthkapsel bei Acidose, bei der Vigantolvergiftung und im Para-Hormonversuch stammen aus seiner Feder, und gemeinsam mit

with six beds for male patients and three for female patients were added and on October 1, 1893, the Clinic for Ear-, Nose- and Throat-Diseases at the University of Graz was opened. Gradually, HABERMANN was able to enlarge the department, but it took until 1913 before he could move into the new clinic with sixty beds and all other necessary service-rooms. At the beginning, only one assistant and one secondary physician were employed, to whom a second assistant was added in 1903. In 1899 HABERMANN became "titular" professor and in 1913 full professor. With his research on occupational deafness of a brazier he became a pioneer in this field of medicine. According to MESSERKLINGER, "it was without doubt a prophetical deed of HABERMANN to prove anatomically how detrimental noise can be to the ear. Since then the detrimental effect of noise on other organs has been ascertained."[71] HABERMANN was also able to prove the beginning of cholesteatoma due to immigration of the epidermis into the middle ear.[72]

From the very beginning HABERMANN also lectured on diseases of the nose and pharynx, whereas laryngology remained within the field of internal medicine. During the winter term of the year 1895/96 HABERMANN gave a series of lectures on "Clinic of Diseases of the Ear" and also on "Clinic of Diseases of the Nose and Throat". During the summer term of 1896 he lectured on "Clinic of Diseases of the Nose, Pharynx and Larynx", thereby uniting the specialties.[73]

HABERMANN trained a large number of students among whom we find such excellent otologists as Otto BARNICK, Karl BAUERREISS, Karl BIEHL, Max KRASSNIG, Otto MAYER, Erich PHLEPS, and Walter STUPKA.

When HABERMANN retired in 1922, Johannes ZANGE (1880–1969; M. D. 1907 [Halle], lecturer 1913 [Jena], associate professor 1919 [Jena]) received a call to Graz. At that time ZANGE had already completed a period of fruitful scientific work. In 1919 his monograph "Pathological Anatomy and Physiology of Inflammation of the Labyrinth Originating in the Middle Ear" had appeared. This work was the result of many years of consequent and systematic research. Already as a student of pathological anatomy ZANGE had directed his attention to the changes in the labyrinth of the ear. Later he continued his research in this field and also made it the topic of his *"Habilitation"*. With the above-mentioned monograph ZANGE "showed the way of conservative and operative treatment of inflammations of the labyrinth and its secondary diseases in the skull."[74] During his first years in Graz ZANGE devoted himself to the research on oto- and rhinogenous meningitis including traumatic meningitis.

Gustav HOFER (1887–1970) succeeded ZANGE in Graz when the latter received a call to Jena in 1931. It was HOFER who suggested to F. X. KOCH to study the advantageous influence of male sexual hormones for treating senile deafness. HOFER's work is best described by his successor at the Graz Clinic, Walter MESSERKLINGER: "In 1913 HOFER became operating surgeon at the Clinic EISELSBERG. During the First World War he served as physician on the front-line, and was later transferred to the surgical company of EISELSBERG. Later he was appointed head of a large military infirmary. Later he became first assistant at the Clinic of Laryngology and Rhinology of Markus HAJEK. In this position HOFER played a leading role in the development of our specialty by introducing a number of major improvements and surgery of the larynx was further developed. Colleagues from all over the

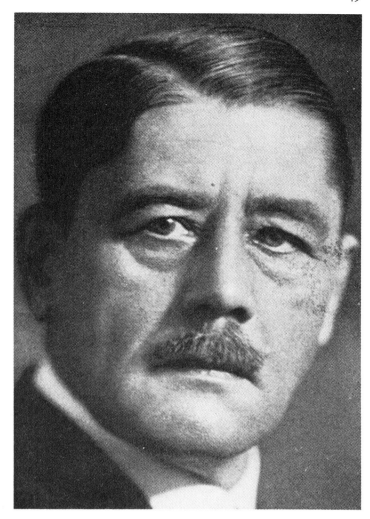

Heinrich Herzog

F. J. LANG beschrieb er die Krankheitszeichen der chronischen Tonsillitis. Auch die bösartigen Geschwülste des Kehlkopfes und der Speiseröhre beschäftigten ihn; den Nebenhöhlenerkrankungen widmete er zahlreiche Publikationen.
Im März 1943, nach KRAINZ' frühem Tod, stand die Fakultät vor der schwierigen Frage der Neubesetzung der Klinik. Die Welt stand in Flammen, und Wirrnisse jeder Art beeinträchtigten das akademische Leben, die auch zu KRAINZ' Lebzeiten schon die Geschehnisse an den Universitäten, aber auch das Leben in Österreich insgesamt belasteten. Der Reichsminister für Wissenschaft, Erziehung und Volksbildung ernannte am 17. November 1943 Werner KINDLER (1895–1970) zum neuen Vorstand der Klinik. KINDLER betreute die Klinik bis zum Juni 1945; nach ihm wurde sie zunächst von W. STRIKKER kommissarisch geleitet.
Am 30. Oktober 1945 wurde Ludwig HÖRBST zum neuen Vorstand der Ohren-, Nasen-, Halsklinik berufen. Mit 19. März 1954 erfolgte seine Ernennung zum Ordinarius. Nach Beseitigung der größten Schwierigkeiten und dem Anlaufen der ersten Reorganisationsmaßnahmen normalisierte sich das alltägliche Leben an der Klinik wieder so weit, daß die notwendigen Kontakte mit den Fachkliniken des In- und Auslandes hergestellt werden konnten. Ein Verdienst HÖRBSTS, über das wir ihn selbst zu Wort kommen lassen, sei speziell hervorgehoben, nämlich die Errichtung der Lehrkanzel für Audiologie und Phoniatrie im Jahr 1968, zu deren Vorstand Walter SCHLORHAUFER (geb. 1920) ernannt wurde. Mit dieser Lehrkanzel „tritt die Ohren-, Nasen-, Halsklinik Innsbruck wieder in eine neue Phase ihrer Entwicklung ein. Es steht zu hoffen, daß diese Akzentsetzung ihr jene Weite des Blickes verleiht, die notwendig ist, um einer Zukunft gewachsen zu sein, die vor ihr liegt."[77] Heinrich SPOENDLIN (geb. 1927 in Zürich) wurde als Nachfolger von Ludwig HÖRBST berufen. SPOENDLINS Hauptarbeitsgebiet ist die experimentelle Pathologie und die elektronenmikroskopischen Untersuchungen der Feinstruktur des Innenohres.
Hatte noch Viktor URBANTSCHITSCH in WIEN lediglich „Klinik der Ohrenkrankheiten" gelesen, so kündigte Heinrich NEUMANN gleich in seinem ersten Semester, dem Sommersemester 1919, „Nasen-, Ohren- und Kehlkopfkrankheiten" an und seit dem Wintersemester 1919/20 „Klinik der Ohren-, Nasen- und Kehlkopfkrankheiten". Die Entwicklung des Faches nach NEUMANNS erzwungenem Rücktritt skizziert Kurt BURIAN (geb. 1921), seit 1970 Vorstand der II. Universitätsklinik für Hals-, Nasen- und Ohrenkrankheiten in Wien: „Zur Zeit der Begründung dieses Faches (1873) wurde von den ersten Ordinarien (GRUBER und POLITZER) die Ohrenheilkunde betrieben und von SCHRÖTTER VON KRISTELLI in anderen Räumlichkeiten des Allg. Krankenhauses die Laryngologie. Diese fachliche Trennung hat sich weitgehend bis zur Mitte der 30er Jahre erhalten. Sie kam unter anderem auch in der Bezeichnung zum Ausdruck: ‚Klinik für Ohren-Nasen-Kehlkopfkrankheiten' und Klinik für ‚Hals-Nasen-Ohrenkrankheiten'. So galt in der Vorkriegszeit HAJEK als Begründer der modernen Rhinologie und NEUMANN als der führende Otologe. Beide haben sich zwar auch mit den jeweils anderen Gebieten befaßt, aber eben nur am Rande. Ihre Schwerpunkte waren entweder die Erkrankungen der Nase und des Kehlkopfes oder jene des Ohres, sie haben aber immerhin durch namhafte Vertreter des jeweiligen Gegenfaches dies an ihren Kliniken vertreten und bis zu einem gewissen Grad gefördert.

world came to Vienna, which at this time was the center of laryngology. This was also the period when rhino-laryngology was united with otology. In 1931 HOFER accepted a call to Graz and stayed there until his retirement in 1959. He fully devoted himself to basic research in rhino-laryngology as well as to the unification of otology with rhino-laryngology."[75]
In INNSBRUCK no lectures in otology or laryngology were given until 1892. We may assume that instruction in otology and laryngology, if at all, was given by internal specialists or surgeons.
In 1893 Georg JUFFINGER (1853–1913) was appointed associate professor of rhinology, laryngology and otiatry. In 1894 the Clinic of Otology at the University of Innsbruck was established. At that time the clinic consisted merely of six beds and working conditions must have been extremely difficult. This is also attested by Ludwig HÖRBST (1903–1981).[76] JUFFINGER, born in Hötting near Innsbruck, became M. D. in 1881 and lecturer in otology in Vienna in 1892. Until his call to Innsbruck in 1911 he was assistant to SCHRÖTTER and his successor STOERK. According to his training, JUFFINGER was a laryngologist, although he also devoted himself to otology. Scientifically he conducted research on scleroma and tuberculosis of the mucosa of the larger air-passages.
After JUFFINGER's death in 1914, Karl GUGLER acted as substitute chairman of the clinic. In 1916 Heinrich HERZOG (1875–1938) became chairman.
Born in Pfaffenburg (Bavaria), HERZOG studied medicine in Munich and Würzburg and received his M. D. in 1900. In 1915 he became associate professor. His call to Innsbruck came during his war service. HERZOG especially devoted himself to experimental labyrinthitis. Apart from his research work, his energies went into the re-establishment and reorganization of the Innsbruck clinic. Although he was able to enlarge his department, the lack of room finally made him leave Innsbruck for Munich in 1928.
In 1931 Wilfried KRAINZ (1895–1943), then associate professor, was appointed head of the clinic. KRAINZ' main scientific work was on pneumatization and inflammatory diseases of the mastoid process. He also published experimental and histological studies on changes of the labyrinth capsule of animals caused by acidosis, vigantol poisoning and in para-hormone-experiment. Together with F. J. LANG he described the symptoms of chronic tonsillitis. Other works of KRAINZ are devoted to malignant tumors of the larynx and the esophagus.
KRAINZ' death in 1943, during World War Two, brought about the difficult task of appointing his successor in Innsbruck. On November 17, 1943, Werner KINDLER (1895–1970) was appointed as KRAINZ' successor. KINDLER headed the clinic until June 1945, followed for a short time by W. STRICKER. On October 30, 1945, Ludwig HÖRBST was appointed Head of the Clinic of Otology, Rhinology and Laryngology, but only in 1954 did he become full professor. HÖRBST immediately started with the reconstruction and reorganization of the clinic. He must be given particular credit for establishing the Clinic of Audiology and Phoniatry in Innsbruck in 1968. Walter SCHLORHAUFER became its head. "This clinic will bring about a new period in the development of the Innsbruck University Clinic of Oto-Rhino-Laryngology. We hope that by adding this new clinic we will be able to enlarge our focus, for only this seems to be the right direction for future developments."[77]

In der Zeit nach 1938 mit all ihren politischen und rassischen Konsequenzen kam es zu einer weiteren Verschmelzung der Fachbereiche an beiden Kliniken. UNTERBERGER – ein ZANGE-Schüler und Allrounder – übernahm [1939] die I. Hals-, Nasen- und Ohrenklinik und hat an der ehemaligen ‚Ohrenklinik' das ganze Fach und auch an der II. HNO-Klinik wurde unter WESSELY die gesamte Hals-Nasen-Ohrenheilkunde betrieben. Es war dies für den damaligen Stand des Faches sicherlich die einzig richtige Entwicklung. UNTERBERGER schloß sich 1945 der sich zurückziehenden deutschen Wehrmacht an und gelangte so nach Kärnten, wo er Anfang 1946 das Primariat für Hals-, Nasen- und Ohrenheilkunde am Landeskrankenhaus Klagenfurt übernahm.
... Nachfolger UNTERBERGERS in Wien wurde [1945] Emil SCHLANDER, ein ganz ausgezeichneter Ohrchirurg, der gemeinsam mit seinen Mitarbeitern gleichfalls das ganze Fach vertreten hat. ...
An der II. Hals-Nasen-Ohrenklinik wurde [1945] Prof. WIETHE Vorstand. Er hat als Schüler HAJEKS besonders die Rhino-Laryngologie vertreten; ... Seine nur 4jährige Tätigkeit reichte nicht aus, eine Schule aufzubauen. In dem folgenden Interregnum führte KOSCHIER als kommissarischer Leiter die Klinik.
1953 übernahm nochmals WESSELY die Klinik; doch nur ein Jahr nach seiner Berufung verstarb er plötzlich. Erst mit seinem Nachfolger NOVOTNY, 1. Oberarzt von SCHLANDER, begannen [1955] für die II. HNO-Klinik wieder ruhige Zeiten; er leitete die Klinik durch 27 Jahre.
Nach SCHLANDERS Emeritierung wurde ich im Jahr 1959 supplierender Leiter der I. Hals-Nasen-Ohrenklinik, damals eine Klinik mit über 100 Betten.... In den 60er Jahren ergaben sich durch die notwendig gewordene Installierung einer neurochirurgischen Klinik Raumschwierigkeiten. Es war naheliegend, diese durch die Auflösung der vakanten I. HNO-Klinik und Verwendung deren Räume zu lösen.
... Der nun stillgelegten I. Hals-Nasen-Ohrenklinik verblieben lediglich ein größeres Krankenzimmer und die Ambulanzräume; sie wurde zur Filialstation der II. Hals-Nasen-Ohrenklinik erklärt und hatte die Aufgabe, ambulante Patienten und die Konsiliarfälle des alten Allg. Krankenhauses zu betreuen. ...
Nach Reaktivierung der stillgelegten Klinik [1969] wurden über Wunsch von NOVOTNY die Namen geändert, so daß die im neuen Allgemeinen Krankenhaus gelegene Klinik als I., jene im alten Haus als II. HNO-Klinik bezeichnet wurde. Durch die Bemühungen von Prof. LINDNER gab es ab 1970 wieder eine II. HNO-Klinik, ... Erst 1972 konnte ein eigener Bau errichtet werden, der die neurootologische, die phoniatrische Abteilung, die Audiologie und das klinikeigene Rechenzentrum aufnahm."[78]
Kurt BURIAN hat die Evoked Response Audiometry (ERA, BERA) und die objektive Sprachaudiometrie entwickelt. Weiters wurde von ihm mit der Technischen Universität Wien die „Wiener Hörprothese" zur Rehabilitation bei Taubheit ausgearbeitet.

HÖRBST was succeeded by Heinrich SPOENDLIN (born in 1927 in Zurich) whose main field of work is experimental pathology and research of the finer structures of the inner ear by means of electron microscope.
Whereas Viktor URBANTSCHITSCH had lectured only on "Clinic of Ear Diseases" in Vienna, Heinrich NEUMANN already in his first semester as head of the clinic in 1919 lectured on "Diseases of the Nose, Ear and Larynx" and during the winter term of the year 1919/20 on "Clinic of Diseases of the Ear, Nose and Larynx". The development of the specialty after NEUMANN's forced retirement is described by Kurt BURIAN (born in 1921), who since 1970 has headed the Second University Clinic for Throat-, Nose- and Ear-Diseases in Vienna: "When the specialty was founded in 1873, the first professors, GRUBER and POLITZER, devoted themselves solely to otology, while SCHRÖTTER von KRISTELLI practiced laryngology in other rooms of the Vienna General Hospital. Broadly speaking, this separation of the specialties was maintained until the mid-1930s. It was also expressed in the titles 'Clinic for Diseases of the Ear, Nose and Larynx', and 'Clinic for Diseases of the Throat, Nose and Ear'. Before the Second World War HAJEK was regarded as the founder of modern rhinology and NEUMANN as the leading otologist. Both covered the other specialty as well, but only marginally. Their main work was either devoted to diseases of the nose and larynx or the ear, respectively. After 1938 the different specialties were united. UNTERBERGER, a student of ZANGE, was an all-rounder and in 1939 he became head of the First Clinic of Throat-Nose- and Ear-Diseases. He had a complete knowledge of the specialty such as WESSELY had as head of the Second Clinic of ENT-Diseases. This was certainly the best possible development for the specialty then ...
In 1945 UNTERBERGER was succeeded by Emil SCHLANDER, who was an excellent aural surgeon, but also an all-round-specialist ...
In 1945 WIETHE became head of the Second ENT-Clinic. Being a student of HAJEK, he particularly devoted himself to rhino-laryngology ... He headed the clinic only for four years and thus was unable to establish a 'school'. KOSCHIER substituted until, in 1953, WESSELY again became head of the clinic, but died only one year later. NOVOTNY, SCHLANDER's former first head-physician, became head of the Second ENT-Clinic in 1955; a position which he held for 27 years.
When SCHLANDER retired, I was appointed in 1959 to substitute the First ENT-Clinic. At this time the clinic consisted of more than 100 beds ... When in the 60s a new clinic of neurosurgery was established, the lack of space was solved by using the rooms of the First ENT-Clinic, which still did not have a new head ... We were left with one larger sick-room and the out-patient department became part of the Second ENT-Clinic ... In 1969 the clinic was re-activated and the names were changed: the former Second ENT-Clinic became now the first one and vice versa. Due to Professor LINDNER's efforts a Second ENT-Clinic was re-established in 1970 ... Only in 1972 was a new building added, which houses the departments of neuro-otology, phoniatry, audiology, and the computer station of our clinic."[78]
Kurt BURIAN developed Evoked Response Audiometry (ERA, BERA) and objective speech audiometry. In collaboration with Vienna's Technical University he developed the "Viennese Auditory Prothesis" for the rehabilitation of deaf people.

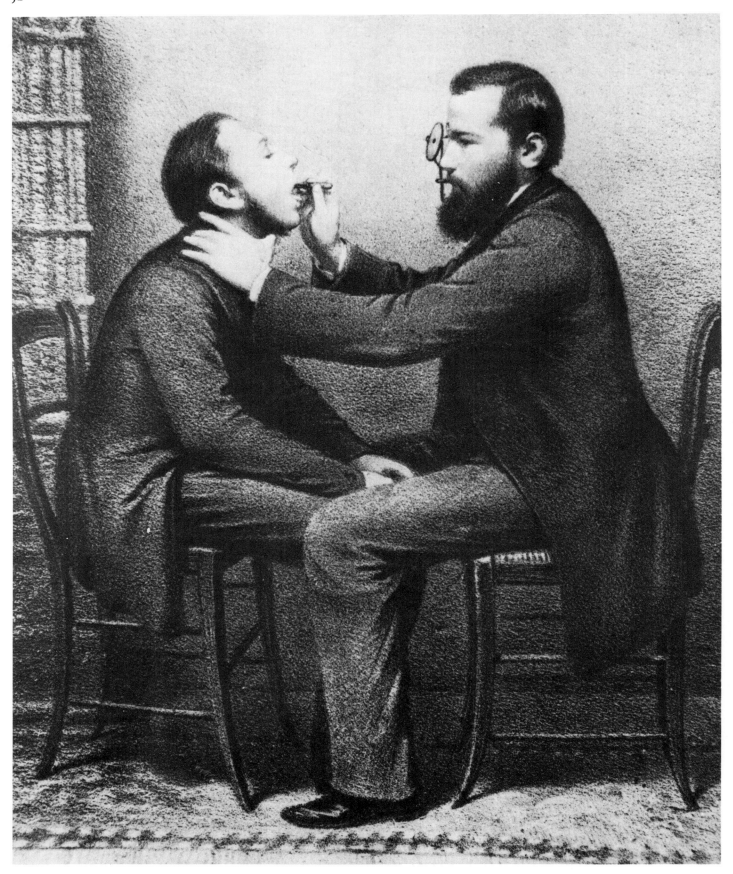

DIE LARYNGOLOGEN UND DIE RHINOLOGEN
THE LARYNGOLOGISTS AND RHINOLOGISTS

Die physikalische Diagnostik hatte indirekt über das normale und krankhafte Geschehen im Brustraum Auskunft gegeben; sie wurde in der zweiten Hälfte des 18. und zu Beginn des 19. Jahrhunderts in Österreich von Leopold VON AUENBRUGGER (1722–1809) und in Frankreich von René Theophile Hyacinthe LAENNEC (1781–1826) entwickelt. Dann wurden immer häufiger und tauglicher Versuche unternommen, die einen direkten Einblick in den Organismus gestatten sollten. Verschiedene, z. T. recht monströse Apparate zeigen, wie man zu Beginn und in der Mitte des 18. Jahrhunderts bestrebt war, Licht in die Körperhöhlen zu spiegeln.
Da machten Ludwig TÜRCK (1810–1868) und Johann Nepomuk CZERMAK (1828–1873) die Laryngoskopie im Jahr 1858 der Klinik dienstbar. Diese neue Methode der Spiegelbetrachtung mit von außen reflektiertem Licht setzte sich in kurzer Zeit durch und eroberte von Wien aus die Welt, sodaß Leopold SCHRÖTTER VON KRISTELLI (1837–1908) in seiner „Festrede, gelegentlich der TÜRCK-CZERMAK Gedenkfeier und des fünfzigjährigen Bestehens des Kehlkopfspiegels", die er als Ehrenpräsident des ersten internationalen Laryngo-Rhinologen Kongresses in Wien im Jahr 1908 hielt, nicht übertrieb, wenn er sagte: „Wenn ich das Verlassen des philosophisch-spekulativen Standpunktes und die Einkehr zur naturwissenschaftlichen Methode als das wichtigste Ereignis des vorigen Jahrhunderts im Werdegange der Medizin ansehe, so möchte ich unter den bedeutendsten Errungenschaften, die aus diesem Boden hervorgegangen sind – der Erfindung des Augenspiegels, dem Verfahren, Medikamente auf subkutanem Wege dem Organismus einzuverleiben, der Anti- und Asepsis, der Entwicklung der Bakteriologie, der Einführung der Serum- und Organotherapie, letztere beruhend auf der Erkenntnis der inneren Sekretion, und endlich der Radiologie – als eine ebenbürtige Schöpfung den Kehlkopfspiegel bezeichnen. Es soll nun meine Aufgabe sein, den Platz festzustellen, welchen die aus der Erfindung des Kehlkopfspiegels hervorgegangene, bald zu einem abgerundeten Wissenszweige herangewachsene Larynologie im Verlauf der ersten 50 Jahre ihres Bestehens unter den übrigen Disziplinen der Medizin gewonnen hat."[79]
Folgen wir also der Darstellung SCHRÖTTERS: Seit dem Sommer 1857 hatte Ludwig TÜRCK, ohne Kenntnis der Erfindung des spanischen Gesangslehrers Manuel GARCIA, der damals in London 1854 mit einem Spiegelchen zu stimmphysiologischen Zwecken seinen eigenen Kehlkopf besichtigt und die Ergebnisse seiner Untersuchungen im Jahr 1855 publiziert hat, zuerst an Leichen und dann an Patienten seiner Abteilung, der Nerven- und 6. Medizinischen Abteilung des Allgemeinen Krankenhauses, mittels des Sonnenlichtes mit dem von ihm konstruierten Kehlkopfspiegel laryngoskopiert, eifrig Befunde gesammelt, bis eben das mangelnde Sonnenlicht im Winter seine Arbeit unterbrach.
Im darauffolgenden Frühjahr aber veröffentlichte ein anderer, nämlich der aus Prag gebürtige Physiologe Johann Nepomuk CZERMAK (1828–1873) in der „Wiener Medizinischen

Physical diagnostics indirectly provided evidence of the normal as well as pathological processes taking place in the thorax. It was developed in the second half of the 18th and at the beginning of the 19th century in Austria by Leopold von AUENBRUGGER (1722–1809) and in France by René Theophile Hyacinthe LAENNEC (1781–1826). Attempts to directly look into the cavities of the body followed and proved successful. Numerous and very often monstrous instruments dating back to the beginning and the middle of the 18th century give evidence of this bold undertaking. In 1858 Ludwig TÜRCK (1810–1868) and Johann Nepomuk CZERMAK (1828–1873) made laryngoscopy serve clinical practice. Within a very short period of time this new method of using a little laryngeal mirror to carry out laryngoscopies by means of reflected light became popular and from Vienna went around the globe. Therefore, Leopold SCHRÖTTER VON KRISTELLI (1837–1903) in his "Festive Address on the Occasion of the TÜRCK-CZERMAK-Commemoration" held at the First International Congress of Laryngo-Rhinologists in Vienna in 1908, did not exaggerate when stating: "In my opinion the most important event of the last century in the field of medicine was the abandonment of the philosophical speculative point of view and the turn toward scientific methods. Concerning scientific methods I would place the invention of the laryngoscope in its importance next to the invention of the ophthalmoscope, subcutaneous injections, anti- and asepsis, the development of bacteriology, the introduction of serum and organotherapy, the latter of which is based on the knowledge of the inner secretion, and radiology. – In my lecture I will try to define the position of laryngology among the other medical specialties in the course of the past fifty years; a position which is based on the invention of the laryngoscope."[79] – Let us now follow SCHRÖTTER's account: In 1854 the Spanish vocal music teacher Manuel GARCIA had inspected his own larynx for vocal-physiological purposes by means of a little mirror, and in 1855 published his "Observations on the Human Voice" in the 'Proceedings of the Royal Society of London' (7,399–410). Unaware of GARCIA's invention, Ludwig TÜRCK occupied himself in the wards of the Vienna General Hospital during the summer of 1857 with the little laryngeal mirror he had constructed himself and carried out laryngoscopies by means of sunlight on the patients of his department. TÜRCK carried on with his research until the lack of sunlight interrupted his work. In the following spring someone else, the Prague-born physiologist Johann Nepomuk CZERMAK published his observations which he had made on his own larynx with the aid of artificial light in the previous winter by using the mirror he had borrowed from TÜRCK in the "Vienna Medical Weekly".[80] "Herr TÜRCK simply always came too late", CZERMAK stated laconically, but this time he was wrong: Whereas in his discovery of the principle of secondary degeneration, about which TÜRCK had informed the Society of Physicians on November 29, 1849, he had been beaten by the Englishman A. V. WALLER by exactly one week – the

Wochenschrift' seine, am eigenen Kehlkopf während des vergangenen Winters bei künstlicher Beleuchtung mit dem von TÜRCK entlehnten Spiegelchen gemachten Beobachtungen.[80] – „Herr Türck kam eben immer zu spät", stellte CZERMAK lakonisch fest, irrte dieses Mal aber. War TÜRCK im Falle der Entdeckung des Prinzips der sekundären Degeneration der Engländer A. V. WALLER um genau eine Woche zuvorgekommen und war ihm Ähnliches mit seinen Versuchen zur Feststellung der Folgen von Halbseitenläsion des Rückenmarks widerfahren (dabei war ihm BROWN-SÉQUARD zuvorgekommen), so „versuchte sich diesmal der Zauderer in jener denkwürdigen Sitzung der Gesellschaft der Ärzte am 9. April 1858 seinen Prioritätsanspruch zu sichern. Am 14. April erkannte ihn auch CZERMAK ausdrücklich an; in späteren Publikationen aber zog er diese Anerkennung zurück. Der Prioritätsstreit zwischen TÜRCK und CZERMAK, der ‚TÜRCKENKRIEG', hatte begonnen. Sicherlich war er für den eigentlichen Erfinder sehr schmerzvoll, für den neuen Wissenschaftszweig aber höchst nützlich. Schlagartig eroberte sich die Laryngologie die medizinische Welt. Der schwerfällig produzierende, äußerungsgehemmte TÜRCK hatte in dem welt- und redegewandten CZERMAK einen außerordentlich expeditiven, versuchserfahrenen Rivalen gefunden, der im ersten Ansatz viele technische, methodische und therapeutische Möglichkeiten des neuen Verfahrens, künstliche Beleuchtung, Rhinoskopie und laryngoskopische Kontrolle lokaltherapeutischer Eingriffe, teils selbst entwickelte, teils anbahnte. Im Agon der beiden Männer blühte das neue Fach der Laryngologie in erstaunlich kurzer Zeit mächtig empor"[81], schreibt Erna LESKY. Zug um Zug erfolgten Publikation und Gegenpublikation: Auf CZERMAKS Mitteilungen vom 27. März und 17. April folgte eine Entgegnung TÜRCKS als „Schluss einer grösseren Abhandlung über den Kehlkopfrachenspiegel und seine Anwendung bei Krankheiten des Kehlkopfes und seiner Umgebung, aus Nr. 25 und 26 vom 21. und 28. Juni 1859 der ‚allgemeinen Wiener medizinischen Zeitung' besonders abgedruckt." Dort heißt es abschließend in Sperrdruck: „Wenn also LISTON schon im Jahre 1840 vorschlug, sich beim Glottisödem zur Untersuchung eines ähnlichen kleinen Spiegels zu bedienen, wie ihn die Zahnärzte in Gebrauch haben, und GARCIA mittelst eines ähnlichen Spiegels Untersuchungen über die Stimmbildung anstellte, so ist die neuerliche Anregung zur praktischen Verwerthung des Kehlkopfspiegels und die Umwandlung des bisher nur ganz ausnahmsweise vertragenen Instrumentes in ein brauchbares, durch eine beträchtliche Anzahl bekannt gemachter pathologischer Fälle bereits bewährtes diagnostisches Hilfsmittel mein, und nicht Herrn CZERMAK's Werk, indem letzterer nur die von mir bereits seit länger ins Werk gesetzte Idee in ganz unberechtigter Weise ohne meine Zustimmung veröffentlichte, und nachträglich meine Priorität in der klarsten Weise selbst anerkannte, während er keine praktisch brauchbare Methode des laryngoskopischen Verfahrens anzugeben im Stande war." Auf CZERMAKS Veröffentlichung von sieben pathologisch-laryngologischen Fällen – wir dürfen bei dieser Darstellung wieder Erna LESKY folgen – folgte am 20. Februar 1859 jene TÜRCKS vom 14. März, gleichfalls sieben Fälle umfassend. Anfang 1860 erschien CZERMAKS Broschüre „Der Kehlkopfspiegel und seine Verwerthung für Physiologie und Medicin" in Leipzig, Ende 1860 TÜRCKS „Praktische Anleitung zur Laryngoskopie" in Wien. „Beide wurden ins Französische übersetzt, die TÜRCKS natürlich später (1861) als die principle of secondary degeneration became known in medical history as the "law of Wallerian degeneration" –, and similarly in his research on hemilateral lesion, about which he reported to the Society of Physicians on November 14, 1850, while BROWN-SÉQUARD had already published his experiments on March 2, 1850, this time, however, "the procrastinator (TÜRCK) asserted his claim to priority in a memorable session of the Society of Physicians on April 9, 1858. On April 14, CZERMAK definitely acknowledged TÜRCK's claim, but he withdrew the acknowledgment in subsequent publications. Thus began the priority dispute between TÜRCK and CZERMAK, nicknamed 'The Turckish War.' This dispute was undoubtedly very painful for the actual inventor, but most useful for the new branch of science. Laryngology promptly conquered the medical world. To TÜRCK, who was slow in his work and lacked ease of expression, the adroit and eloquent CZERMAK was an extraordinarily resourceful and experienced rival, who himself at the very beginning partly developed and partly initiated many technical methodological and therapeutic potentialities of the new process, artificial lighting, rhinoscopy and laryngoscopic control of local treatment. Under the impetus of the intense dispute between the two men, the new subject of laryngology developed greatly in an amazingly short period of time."[81] Publications and counterpublications followed one another. CZERMAK's communications of March 27 and April 17, 1858, were, among others, followed by TÜRCK's "Conclusion of a Larger Treatise Concerning the Laryngo-rhinoscope and its Application for Diseases of the Larynx and Neighbouring Parts" in numbers 25 and 26 of the "Vienna General Medical Journal" of June 21 and 28, 1859. In this article TÜRCK concludes: "Although LISTON as early as 1840 suggested the use of a small mirror, which was used by dentists, for the study of larynx oedema, and GARCIA used a similar instrument for vocal-physiological purposes, the new impulse for the practical use of the laryngeal mirror and its transformation from an instrument that could hardly be tolerated by patients when inserted into a useful instrument for diagnostic purposes, is solely my and not Mr. CZERMAK's achievement. The latter only published – without my authorization – my observations without my knowledge or consent. He later clearly acknowledged my priority claims, while he himself was unable to specify a practically useful method of the laryngoscopic procedure." CZERMAK's publication on February 20, 1859, of seven pathologic-laryngologic cases was followed by TÜRCK's publication on March 14, which also covered seven cases. At the beginning of 1860 – as Erna LESKY reports – CZERMAK's booklet "On the Laryngoscope and its Employment in Physiology and Medicine" appeared in Leipzig, and TÜRCK's "Practical Guide to Laryngoscopy" appeared in Vienna at the end of 1860. "Both these works were translated into French, TÜRCK's (1861) later, of course, than CZERMAK's (June 1860). The latter had already also appeared in English in 1861 when TÜRCK's 'Clinical Research on Different Diseases of the Larynx, Trachea and Pharynx' was published by William and Norgate in London in 1862. 'Herr TÜRCK simply always came too late',"[82] writes Erna LESKY. Starting in 1858, CZERMAK traveled frequently: in Germany, France and Great Britain he propagated the new science. This is also the reason why for some time CZERMAK was regarded as the true founder of laryngology, who "acquired enthusiastic disciples everywhere. RUETE, TRAUBE, VOLTOLINI, BATAILLE, Ch. FAUVEL, Morell MACKENZIE and

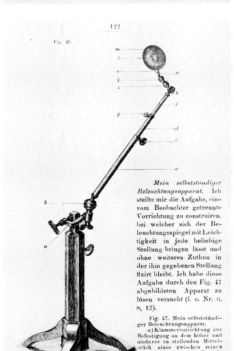

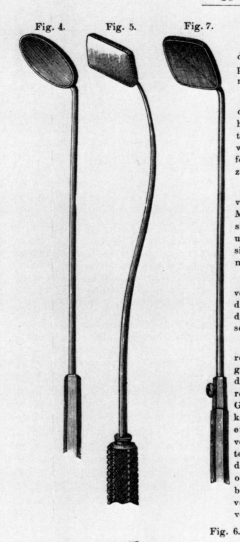

30

Die folgenden Abbildungen mögen dazu dienen, die successiven Metamorphosen dieses Spiegels anschaulich zu machen.

Fig. 4. Halb-Profilansicht meines in der am 26. Juni 1858 erschienenen Abhandlung (5. Beilage) bekannt gemachten Kehlkopfrachenspiegels. Der Spiegel wurde zum leichtern Vergleich mit den folgenden in Halb-Profilansicht gezeichnet.

Fig. 5. Czermak's Kehlkopfspiegel veröffentlicht am 5. März 1859 (Wien. Med. Wochenschr. Nr. 10). Derselbe besitzt schon statt des Drahtes einen Stiel und einen hölzernen Griff, auch nähert sich die Neigung des Spiegels zum Stiel meinem Ansatzwinkel.

Fig. 6. Czermak's Kehlkopfspiegel veröffentlicht 1860 in seiner Monographie des Kehlkopfspiegels und später in der französischen und englischen Uebersetzung derselben.

Fig. 7. Derselbe Spiegel zur grösseren Deutlichkeit und zum leichteren Vergleich mit Fig. 4 in natürlicher Grösse dargestellt. Auf diesen Spiegel sind bereits der gerade Stiel, der gerade hölzerne Griff, der Ansatzwinkel meines Kehlkopfrachenspiegels übertragen, so dass er beinahe eine Copie dieses letzteren vorstellt. Die ganz unwesentlichen Unterscheidungsmerkmale bestehen darin, dass der eigentliche Spiegel anstatt rund oder oval zu sein, vier abgerundete Ecken besitzt, wodurch er nur etwas schwerer vertragen wird, und dass sich der Griff vom Stiel abschrauben lässt[1]).

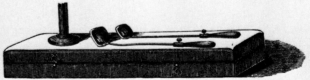

Fig. 6.

¹) Diese ausführliche Darlegung konnte um so weniger unterbleiben, als Czermak (Virch. Arch. und Kehlkopfsp. p. 4) wörtlich sagt, dass er „Herrn Türck auch bei der Construction seiner eigenen Spiegel nichts abgeguckt hat, sondern seinen eigenen Weg gegangen ist."

Seite 52: Johann N. Czermak laryngoskopiert bei Sonnenlicht.
Aus: Czermak, J. N.: Der Kehlkopfspiegel und seine Verwerthung für Physiologie und Medizin. Leipzig 1860.

Page 52: Johann N. Czermak using his laryngoscope with the aid of sunlight.

Links oben: Apparat zur laryngoskopischen Selbstbeobachtung von J. N. Czermak.
Links unten: Beleuchtungsapparat von L. Türck.

Top left: Czermak's apparatus for autolaryngoscopy and demonstration.
Bottom left: Türck's apparatus for laryngoscopy.

Rechts: Fig. 4 zeigt den von L. Türck verwendeten Kehlkopfspiegel. Daneben Modifikationen von J. N. Czermak.
Aus: Türck, Ludwig: Klinik der Krankheiten des Kehlkopfes und der Luftröhre. . . . Wien, Leipzig, Paris 1866.

Right: Figure 4 shows the laryngeal mirror used by L. Türck. Next to it are modifications devised by J. N. Czermak.

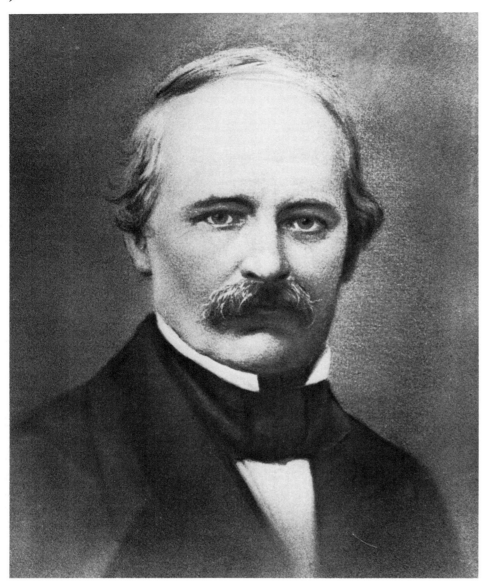

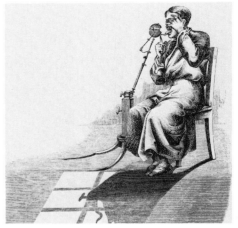

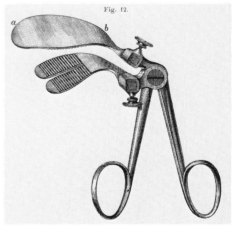

Rechts oben und unten: Autolaryngoskopie bei reflektiertem, direktem Sonnenlicht mit Hilfe eines von Türck konstruierten Zungenhalters (siehe die Abbildung darunter).

Right: Autolaryngoscopy with reflected, direct sunlight by means of a tongue forceps constructed by Türck (shown in the lower picture).

Ludwig Türck hatte seit dem Sommer 1857 mittels des Sonnenlichtes mit dem von ihm konstruierten Kehlkopfspiegel laryngoskopiert. Im darauffolgenden Frühjahr jedoch publizierte Johann Nepomuk Czermak, der während des Winters bei künstlichem Licht mit dem von Türck geborgten und modifizierten Spiegel weitergearbeitet hatte ohne Wissen und Einverständnis Türcks seine Beobachtungen als erster. Der Prioritätsstreit um die Entdeckung des Kehlkopfspiegels fand seinen Niederschlag in einer Reihe einschlägiger Publikationen und bewirkte, daß der neue Wissenschaftszweig, die Laryngoskopie, schlagartig bekannt wurde.

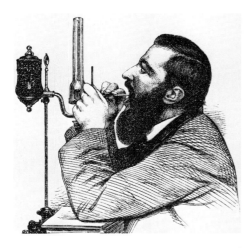

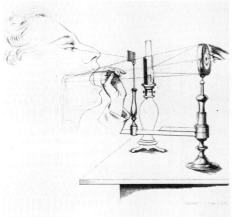

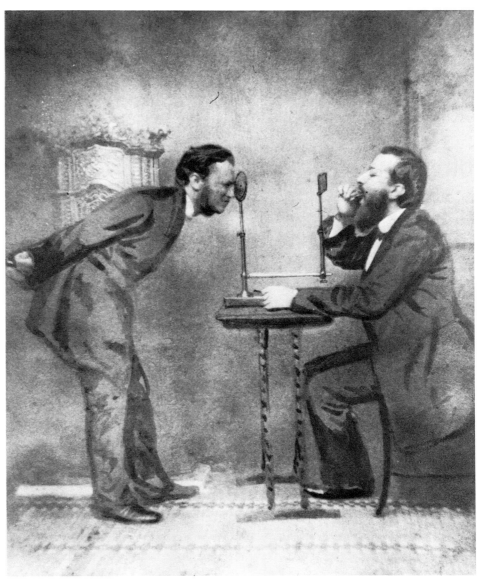

Links oben: Autolaryngoskopie durch J. H. Czermak. Aus: Czermak, Johann N.: Der Kehlkopfspiegel und seine Verwerthung für Physiologie und Medizin. Leipzig 1860.
Links unten: Autolaryngoskopie. Dazu schreibt Czermak: „Ein perspektivisch gezeichnetes Schema meines Verfahrens um vermittelst des Kehlkopfspiegels Beobachtungen anzustellen, ..."

Top left: Autolaryngoscopy. The right hand is holding the laryngeal mirror; the left the flat mirror, represented here only in profile.
Bottom left: Autolaryngoscopic observation and demonstration. From: Czermak, J. N.: On the Laryngoscope and its Employment in Physiology and Medicine. London, 1861.

During the summer of 1857, Ludwig Türck carried out laryngoscopies with a little laryngeal mirror he had constructed himself. He carried on with his research until the lack of sunlight interrupted his work. In the following spring the Prague-born physiologist Johann Nepomuk Czermak published his observations which he had made on his own larynx with the aid of artificial light in the previous winter by using the mirror he had borrowed from Türck. Thus began the priority dispute between Türck and Czermak, which was most useful for the new branch of science, with the result that laryngology promptly became known throughout the world.

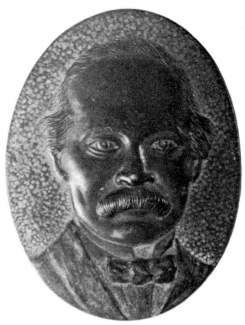 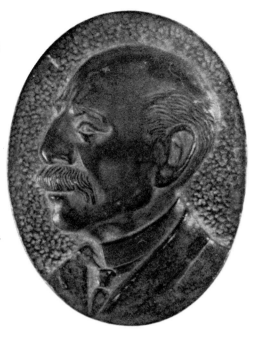

Gedenkplaketten für Ludwig Türck (links) und Johann Nepomuk Czermak (rechts).

Commemorative plaques for Ludwig Türck (left) and Johann Nepomuk Czermak (right).

CZERMAKS (Juni 1860). Diese war bereits 1861 auch in englischer Sprache erschienen, als 1862 Türck mit seinen ‚Clinical Researches on different diseases of the larynx, trachea and pharynx' bei William and Norgate in London herauskam. ‚Herr TÜRCK kam eben immer zu spät.'"[82] Von 1858 an ging CZERMAK auf Reisen nach Deutschland, Frankreich und England und verbreitete überall die Kenntnis der neuen Wissenschaft. Es verwundert daher nicht, daß deshalb eine Zeitlang namentlich im Ausland CZERMAK als der eigentliche Begründer der Laryngologie galt, der auch eine große Zahl von Schülern heranbildete und auch überall „begeisterte Jünger [hinterließ]. RUETE, TRAUBE, VOLTOLINI, BATAILLE, Ch. FAUVEL, Morell MACKENZIE, DURHAM sind nur einige von jenen, die durch CZERMAK zu Pionieren der Laryngo-Rhinologie geworden sind. Ja, auch der Rhinologie! Denn mit seiner Arbeit ‚Über die Inspektion des Cavum pharyngonasale und der Nasenhöhle durch die Choanen vermittelst kleiner Spiegel' hat CZERMAK auch die Rhinologie als neues Spezialgebiet begründet. Einfallsreich und wendig, wie er in der Kombination von Technizismen war, tat er noch ein übriges: Er stellte auch die Photographie und Stereoskopie in den Dienst des jungen Faches. Die drei laryngoskopischen Bilder, die er am 7. November 1861 der Akademie der Wissenschaften vorlegte – sie ruhen heute noch in ihrem Archiv –, sind die ersten stereophotographischen Aufnahmen dieses Organs überhaupt."[83]

Der „TÜRCKENKRIEG", der „die laryngologische Welt lange in Atem hielt", wurde, wie Hermann MARSCHIK feststellt, „endlich in der Weise beigelegt, daß beiden Forschern ihre Verdienste ungeschmälert zuerkannt wurden, wie sie tatsächlich bestanden.... Für uns ist TÜRCK der eigentliche Begründer der wissenschaftlichen Laryngologie als Spezialfach, CZERMAK der Begründer der künstlichen Beleuchtung und der erste Pionier der jungen Wissenschaft, dessen weltgewandtem Wissen und dessen Mitteilungskunst es zu danken ist, daß das Lebenswerk des bescheidenen, in den letzten Jahren sich immer mehr in seine stille Arbeitsklause verschließenden For-

DURHAM are but a few of the men who, owing to CZERMAK, became pioneers of laryngo-rhinology. Yes, rhinology, too. With his publication 'On the Observation of the Cavum Pharyngo-Nasal and of the Nasal Cavity through the Choanae by Means of Small Mirrors', CZERMAK also made the foundation for the specialization of rhinology. Being an inventive and resourceful technician, he also made use of photography and stereoscopy for the benefit of the new subject. The three laryngoscopic pictures which he submitted to the Academy of Sciences on November 7, 1861, and which have been preserved to this day in its archives, were the first stereophotographic pictures ever taken of the larynx."[83] "The Turckish War", which kept laryngology in suspense for a long time, was according to Hermann MARSCHIK finally ended "by attributing to both men their merits as they deserve them: TÜRCK is now credited for having founded laryngology as a specialty and CZERMAK as the founder of laryngoscopy with artificial light and as the first pioneer of the young science, due to whose resourcefulness, eloquence and experience in the ways of the world the specialty conquered the world at least twenty or even thirty years sooner than it otherwise might have." [84] And SCHRÖTTER in his memorial lecture for TÜRCK and CZERMAK stated: "Young physicians would not believe how helpless our patients and we physicians were before the invention of the laryngoscope. Thousands of people died because we were unable to cure them or even relieve their sufferings! How things have changed! Almost every branch of medicine profited greatly by the introduction of the laryngoscope. The study of diseases of the larynx gave rise to new research in the anatomy and physiology of these regions. The results were laid down in valuable publications and new facts were disclosed ... Let us not forget that the introduction of laryngoscopy and more advanced lighting techniques also made it possible to view the oral and the pharyngeal cavities. A thorough study of the sensitivity and localization capacities of the pharynx and larynx was not possible until the laryngoscope enabled an effective

schers in kurzer Zeit in der ganzen Welt bekannt wurde und damit ein junger, heute unentbehrlicher Wissenschaftszweig vielleicht vor dem neuerlichen Versinken in die Vergessenheit bewahrt, sicher aber seine Ausbreitung und Einbürgerung in die Gesamtmedizin des Erdkreises um 20 bis 30 Jahre beschleunigt worden ist."[84] Und SCHRÖTTER sagte in der schon zitierten „Festrede gelegentlich der TÜRCK-CZERMAK-Gedenkfeier": „Kein junger Arzt der Jetztzeit kann sich eine Vorstellung machen von dem Jammerzustande, der in der Zeit vor der Erfindung des Kehlkopfspiegels herrschte, von der beschämenden Hilflosigkeit, in der wir uns dem Kranken gegenüber befanden. Tausende von Menschen sind dahingegangen, denen wir nicht helfen, denen wir nicht einmal eine Erleichterung ihres Leidens bringen konnten! Wie ist dies jetzt ganz anders geworden! Nahezu jede der einzelnen Disziplinen der Medizin wurde durch den Kehlkopfspiegel auf das fruchtbringendste gefördert. Das Studium der Kehlkopfkrankheiten regte neue Forschungen in der Anatomie und Physiologie der bezüglichen Regionen an, welchen wir wertvolle Spezialwerke verdanken und durch die wir eine Reihe wichtiger neuer Tatsachen kennen lernten. . . . Es darf nicht vergessen werden, daß die mit der Einführung der Laryngoskopie gewonnene, bessere Beleuchtung auch der Mund- und Rachenhöhle zugute kam und dadurch alle Vorgänge daselbst gründlicher studiert werden konnten. Erst durch die Spiegel- und die dadurch ermöglichte Sondenuntersuchung war ein genaues Studium der Empfindlichkeit und des Lokalisationsvermögens in der Rachen- und Kehlkopfhöhle möglich."[85]
TÜRCK hat auch – ganz seinem Wesen entsprechend – die große und mühsame Bestandsaufnahme der klinisch-pathologischen Kehlkopfbefunde geleistet und in seiner in Wien bei Braumüller 1866 erschienenen „Klinik der Erkrankung des Kehlkopfes und der Luftröhre" veröffentlicht. Dieses Werk blieb „Jahrzehnte hindurch mit dem dazugehörigen Atlas von ELFINGER und HEITZMANN das Standardwerk des Faches."[86]
In der Vorrede dazu stellt TÜRCK noch einmal mit allem Nachdruck fest: „Die auf Spiegeluntersuchungen gegründeten hier mitgetheilten Thatsachen sind zum größten Theil zuerst von mir aufgefunden worden . . ."[87]
Erst 1861 bekam TÜRCK die Venia legendi und im Jahr 1864 die außerordentliche Professur für Pathologie des Nervensystems und der Stimmorgane; 1868 starb er an Typhus exanthematicus, den er sich an seiner Abteilung geholt hatte. Zwei seiner Schüler – Carl STOERK (1832–1899) und Leopold SCHRÖTTER VON KRISTELLI (1837–1908) – setzten sein Werk fort.
Zwei Jahre nach TÜRCKS Tod wurde 1870 im Quertrakt des Allgemeinen Krankenhauses zwischen dem zweiten und dem siebenten Hof die „Klinik für Laryngoskopie", die erste des Faches in der Welt, geschaffen und Leopold SCHRÖTTER wurde ihr Leiter, nicht aber ihr Vorstand oder Professor.[88] Es spricht für den Weitblick SCHRÖTTERS, daß er schon damals die Entwicklungsmöglichkeiten der Laryngologie erkannte, aber auch für seine Tatkraft und Zielstrebigkeit, daß er nicht nur seine Lehrer Carl VON ROKITANSKY und Joseph SKODA (1805–1881), sondern auch die übrige Fakultät und die Unterrichtsbehörde von der Berechtigung seines Planes zu überzeugen wußte, und es durchsetzte, daß es schon 1870, als er kaum seine Assistentenzeit an der Klinik SKODAS beendet hatte, zur Errichtung der neuen Klinik kam. „Es ist für den Idealismus, den diese Spezialisten-Pioniere – auch die Otologen – aufbrachten, charakteristisch, daß sie jahrzehntelang unentgelt-

examination by probing."[85] As befitted his character, TÜRCK undertook the great and laborious task of establishing the clinical-pathological facts concerning the larynx. In 1866 his "Clinic of the Diseases of the Larynx and the Trachea" appeared in Vienna and, "together with the pertinent atlas by ELFINGER and HEITZMANN, remained the standard work of the subject throughout many decades."[86] In the preface to this work TÜRCK again states: "The facts reported herein and which are based on examinations by means of the laryngoscope, were mainly first discovered by myself."[87]
Only in 1861 did TÜRCK become lecturer "for diseases of the nervous system and of the larynx" and in 1864 he became associate professor. In 1868 he died of typhus exanthematicus which he had acquired in his own department. Two of his disciples – Carl STOERK (1832–1899) and Leopold SCHRÖTTER VON KRISTELLI (1837–1908) – continued his work.
In 1870, two years after TÜRCK's death, the "Clinic of Laryngoscopy", the first one of its kind in the world, was established in the Vienna General Hospital, and Leopold SCHRÖTTER was appointed its head, but was not made full professor.[88] From the very beginning SCHRÖTTER had a clear and accurate conception of the developmental potential inherent in the new specialty. This enabled him – having hardly finished his assistantship at SKODA's clinic – not only to convince his teachers Carl von ROKITANSKY and Joseph SKODA (1805–1881) but the whole medical faculty as well as the ministry of the necessity to establish a clinic of laryngology. "It is characteristic for the idealism of these pioneers of specialization (and the same applies to the otologists) that for decades they worked without a salary, only later maybe decorated with the title 'associate professor' (SCHRÖTTER in 1875). They knew that the all important point at the beginning of the foundation of a specialty was to ensure a place for the practice of their newly founded specialty in the legitimate and representative location of Viennese medicine, the General Hospital, even if the space was extremely limited. This was indeed the case with SCHRÖTTER's clinic: two sickrooms, each with eight beds, and a small chamber for preparations located in the corridor between the second and the seventh court of the General Hospital. But SCHRÖTTER – just as the oculists and otologists – knew how to make best use of the enormous number of ambulatory patients: in 1890 their number had reached some 7,200. By treating these patients the tireless SCHRÖTTER perfected his own knowledge and developed his therapy of stenosis."[89] From 1870 to 1890 SCHRÖTTER headed the laryngological clinic. Like all laryngologists at that time he had received a specialized training in internal medicine. As SKODA's assistant he had learned from his teacher physical diagnostics; from TÜRCK he had learned how to use the laryngoscope and had later perfected himself independently in this new technique. He was a talented teacher who even during his assistantship had held courses in laryngoscopy, and after a short period of time he together with Carl STOERK and Johann SCHNITZLER (1835–1893) made Vienna the center of laryngology. The large number of foreign students who studied laryngology in Vienna made the specialty known in wide circles. "His foreign students were fascinated by the way SCHRÖTTER mixed the languages during his lectures in such a way that it seemed to them as if he spoke three different languages at the same time. Before the discovery of cocaine as a local anaesthetic the removal of a polyp was a major surgical endeavor. The patient had to be prepared for this operation

lich ihre klinischen Leitungsfunktionen ausübten, im Laufe der Zeit geschmückt mit dem Titel eines außerordentlichen Professors (SCHRÖTTER: 1875). Sie wußten, daß in der ersten Aufbauphase alles darauf ankam, ihrem Fach im legitimen Repräsentationsraum der Wiener Medizin, im Allgemeinen Krankenhaus, eine Arbeitsstätte zu erobern. Auch wenn wie im Falle SCHRÖTTERS diese nur aus zwei Krankenzimmern mit 16 Betten und einer kleinen Kammer für Präparate bestand. Umso mehr wußte SCHRÖTTER (wie die Okulisten und Otologen) das reiche Krankengut zu nutzen, das in der Ambulanz zusammenströmte. 1890 waren es bereits 7200 Kranke jährlich. An diesem ‚Material' hat der Unermüdliche sich beharrlich weitergebildet, untersucht, behandelt und seine Stenosentherapie entwickelt."[89] Zwanzig Jahre, von 1870 bis 1890, leitete SCHRÖTTER die laryngologische Klinik. Er ging, wie damals alle Laryngologen, aus der inneren Medizin hervor. Als Assistent SKODAS hatte er von diesem die physikalische Diagnostik der Brustkrankheiten gelernt; bei TÜRCK hatte er das Kehlkopfspiegeln erlernt, sich aber dann autodidaktisch weitergebildet. SCHRÖTTER besaß besondere Freude am Lehren und schon während seiner Assistentenzeit hatte er Kurse in Laryngoskopie abgehalten und bald machte er, zusammen mit Carl STOERK und Johann SCHNITZLER (1835–1893), Wien zum bedeutendsten Zentrum der Laryngologie. Ein großer Zustrom ausländischer Hörer machte das Fach in immer weiteren Kreisen bekannt. „Seine ausländischen Kursisten hat er bezaubert, wenn er die Sprachen so geschickt mischte, daß es ihnen schien, als ob er in dreien zu gleicher Zeit spräche. Eine Polypenentfernung gehörte in der Vor-Kokainära zu den großen operativen Ereignissen. Die Patienten mußten wochenlang vorbereitet werden, um den Eingriff in dem so reflexreichen Raum (Würgen, Husten, Erbrechen) überhaupt zu ertragen. Man kann sich die Bewunderung der Kursteilnehmer vorstellen, als SCHRÖTTER am Ende einer Kursstunde mit einem Polypenquetscher in den Kehlkopf eines Patienten einging und mit eleganter Bewegung das Gewächs seinen Hörern vorführte: ‚Meine Herren, ein großer kaiserlicher königlicher Polyp.'"[90]
Es wurde an der SCHRÖTTERSCHEN Klinik nicht nur die Krankheit exakt festgestellt; sondern unter der Sicht des Kehlkopfspiegels konnte auch operiert werden. SCHRÖTTER hatte einst bei BILLROTHS Vorgänger Franz SCHUH (1804–1865) eine gründliche chirurgische Ausbildung genossen, und war auch durch seine ihm angeborene Geschicklichkeit für operative Eingriffe im Kehlkopf besonders geeignet. Und Geschicklichkeit wurde damals von den Laryngologen im besonderen Maße verlangt! Die Beleuchtungstechnik war noch ganz im Anfangsstadium, und man arbeitete sogar noch mit der Schusterkugel, die zur Verstärkung der Lichtquelle diente und entweder seitlich oder hinter dem Patienten aufgestellt wurde, oft auch hinter dem Operateur. Dann kamen Verbesserungen mit verschiedenen petroleumgespeisten Lampen, dann das Gaslicht, und erst in den achtziger Jahren des vorigen Jahrhunderts kam das Gasglühlicht auf.[91] Auch die Instrumententechnik war noch im Anfangsstadium. Die Hauptschwierigkeit aber lag im Anästhesieproblem, wie Hermann MARSCHIK berichtet: „Obwohl schon TÜRCK eine Methode der Lokalanästhesie mit Morphin-Karbol-Lösung angegeben hatte, wurde diese Methode wegen der starken Reizungen, die sie an der Kehlkopfschleimhaut hervorrief, nicht gern und oft angewendet. So behalf man sich, von Beobachtungen an einzelnen Fällen von Hyp- oder Anästhe-

for several weeks so that he would be able to tolerate the surgical intervention in an area full of reflexes (choking, coughing, vomiting). One may imagine how the participants of SCHRÖTTER'S courses admired the teacher when he, at the end of a lecture, would insert a polypus-forceps into the larynx of a patient and remove the polyp with an elegant movement stating: 'Gentlemen, a large imperial royal polyp.' "[90]
At SCHRÖTTER'S clinic diseases were not only diagnosed exactly, but with the aid of the laryngoscope operations were also performed. SCHRÖTTER had the best possible schooling for performing such operations: he had studied surgical techniques for two years under Franz SCHUH (1804–1865), BILLROTH'S predecessor in Vienna, before starting his specialization. Besides, his manual skill made him especially suited for endolaryngeal operations, for in these days the laryngologists needed skill more than anything else. SCHRÖTTER worked out numerous technical details for examining the larynx and for endolaryngeal operations, such as the concentration of the light in a so-called "Schusterkugel", a glass ball filled with water, which the shoemakers used. It was placed either at the side or behind the patient or even behind the operating physician. Later improvements were made by using kerosene lamps and gas-light; incandescent gas-light was not introduced until the 1880s.[91] Laryngeal instruments for endolaryngeal operations also had to be invented or modified for their special purpose. The main problem, however, was the lack of a suitable anaesthetic, as is reported by Hermann MARSCHIK: "Although TÜRCK had tried to anaesthetize the larynx by using a mixture of acetic morphine, concentrated alcohol and chloroform, this method was not suited for wide-spread use because it caused among other problems general symptoms of intoxication. Therefore, the patients had to be trained for weeks in order to learn gradually how to control the vehement reflexes caused by the insertion of the surgical instrument into the larynx so that spasm of the glottis, a dreaded complication in these days, would not occur. However, very often there was not time enough to train the patient for weeks and get him accustomed to the procedure and the laryngologist could only rely on his own skill if he dared to undertake an endolaryngeal operation. I called this art, which necessitated a sudden, flash-like, however, firm grasp a 'royal' art, which has no parallels in other fields of medicine."[92]
The turning point in laryngology occurred in 1884: Shortly after the death of Eduard JAEGER VON JAXTTHAL (1818–1884), who only in 1883 had become head of the Second University Clinic of Ophthalmology at the Vienna General Hospital, a discovery was made at this clinic, which was not only of great importance for ophthalmology but for surgery in general: the secondary physician Carl KOLLER (1857–1944) discovered that by means of a cocaine solution the cornea of the eye could be anaesthetized. "Perhaps it is not too daring to hope that cocaine will be able to be used successfully as an anaesthetic when removing foreign objects from the cornea or for more major operations, or as a narcotic for retinal or conjunctival diseases."[93] This was the resumé of the preliminary communication read by KOLLER'S friend Josef BRETTAUER (1835–1905) on September 15, 1884, on the occasion of the 16th Congress of German Ophthalmologists in Heidelberg. KOLLER, who had been unable to attend the congress himself because of economic difficulties in the family at that time, had asked BRETTAUER to go there and read KOLLER'S paper "in

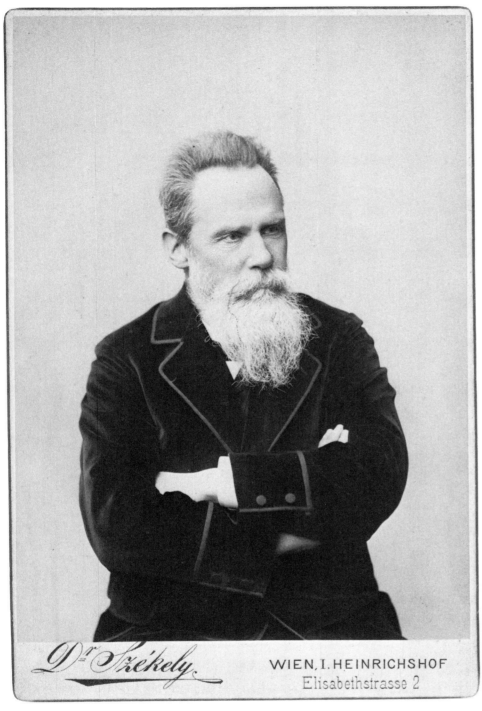
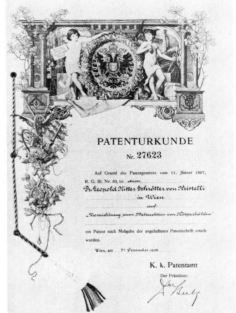
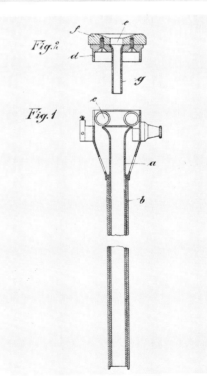

Leopold Schrötter von Kristelli war ein Pionier auf dem Gebiet der Endoskopie der Luftwege. Der ehemalige Skoda-Schüler, Begründer der laryngologischen Klinik in Wien und der Heilanstalt Alland, ließ sich eine „Vorrichtung zum Beleuchten von Körperhöhlen" im Jahr 1906 patentieren.

Leopold Schrötter von Kristelli was a pioneer in endoscopy of the respiratory passages. The former student of Skoda and founder of the Clinic of Laryngology in Vienna and the Sanatorium in Alland took out a patent on his "device to illuminate bodily cavities" in 1906.

62

Leopold Schrötter gemeinsam mit seinen Mitarbeitern in einem Hörsaal des Allgemeinen Krankenhauses.

Leopold Schrötter and his staff in a lecture hall of the Vienna General Hospital.

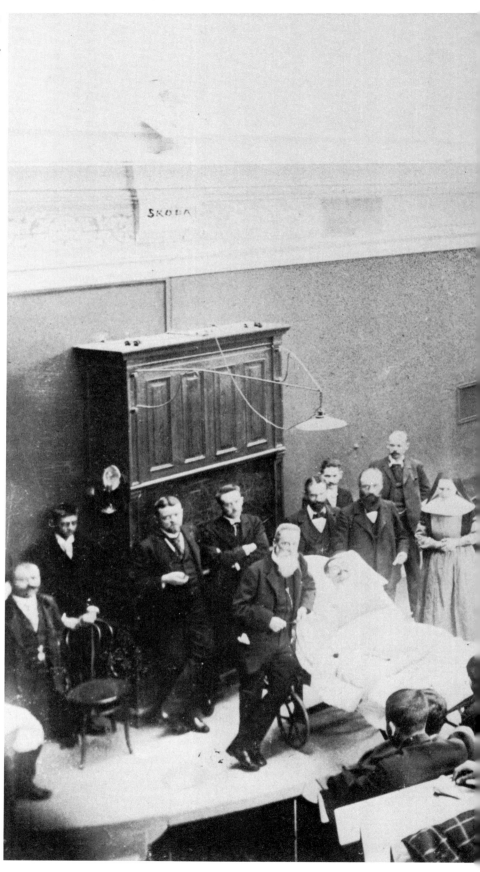

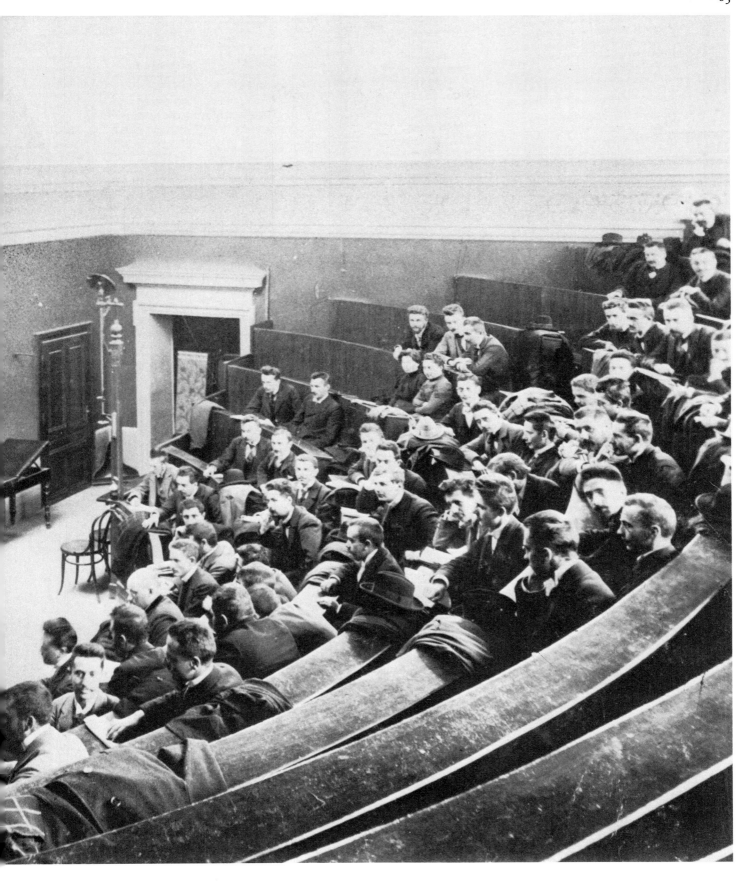

sie des Kehlkopfes ausgehend, mit der Methode der Gewöhnung und Erziehung des Patienten, den heftigen Reflex bei der Einführung eines Instrumentes nach und nach zu meistern und sich trotz Erhaltung der Empfindlichkeit die endolaryngeale Berührung und instrumentelle Manipulation ohne Glottisspasmus gefallen zu lassen. Trotzdem war, von den erwähnten Fällen von Kehlkopfhypästhesie abgesehen, bei aller Mühe eine Anästhesie, wie wir sie heute kennen, kaum zu erreichen. Äußere Gründe drängten soundsooft zur Abkürzung des Verfahrens der Eingewöhnung. Und so blieb dem Laryngologen nichts übrig, als sich auf seine Geschicklichkeit und seine Kunst zu verlassen, wenn er den endolaryngealen Eingriff wagte. Und diese Kunst, die ein blitzartiges und doch sicheres Zugreifen erforderte, ... habe ich ... eine königliche Kunst genannt, die ihresgleichen in keinem anderen der medizinischen Fächer fand."[92]

Die Wende in der Laryngologie erfolgte im Jahr 1884: Unmittelbar nach dem Tode Eduard JAEGERS VON JAXTTHAL (1818–1884), der erst 1883 zum Vorstand der II. Universitäts-Augenklinik im Allgemeinen Krankenhaus in Wien bestellt worden war, wurde in der eben verwaisten Klinik eine Entdeckung gemacht, die nicht nur für die Augenheilkunde von allergrößter Bedeutung war, sondern für alle chirurgischen Fächer: der Sekundararzt Carl KOLLER (1857–1944) stellte fest, daß mit einer Kokainlösung die Oberfläche des Auges unempfindlich gemacht werden könne, so daß nicht nur dem Patienten der Schmerz genommen wurde, sondern auch für den Chirurgen ein wesentlich langsameres und gründlicheres Operieren am Auge möglich wurde. „Vielleicht ist es nicht zu gewagt, wenn ich mich der Hoffnung hingebe, dass das Cocain als Anästheticum bei Entfernung von Fremdkörpern aus der Cornea oder bei größeren Operationen oder als Narkoticum bei Hornhaut- und Conjunctival-Erkrankungen mit Erfolg wird angewendet werden können."[93] Dies teilte KOLLERS Freund Josef BRETTAUER (1835–1905) in einer „Vorläufigen Mitteilung zur Wahrung der Priorität" am 15. September 1884 anläßlich der 16. Versammlung der ophthalmologischen Gesellschaft in Heidelberg der Weltöffentlichkeit mit, da sich KOLLER damals aus finanziellen Gründen eine Reise nach Heidelberg nicht leisten konnte.[94] Später berichtete KOLLER selbst in Wien über seine Entdeckung. Dem damaligen Programm für die Sitzung der Gesellschaft der Ärzte vom 17. Oktober 1884 ist zu entnehmen, daß in Gegenwart des Präsidenten Hofrat VON ARLT (1812–1887), der an diesem Tag den Vorsitz führte, zuerst der Dermatologe Moritz KAPOSI (1837–1902) über einen Fall von Favus universalis sprach und dann am gleichen Abend KOLLER und Leopold KÖNIGSTEIN (1850–1924) über ihre Forschungsergebnisse bei Kokain. Der ursprünglich im Programm auch für diesen Tag vorgesehene Beitrag Edmund JELINEKS (1852–1928) über „Anwendung des Cocains als Anästheticum und Analgeticum an der Schleimhaut des Rachens und des Kehlkopfes" wurde erst eine Woche später in der Gesellschaft der Ärzte, und zwar dann unter dem Vorsitz von Theodor BILLROTH gehalten.

Bereits im Juli 1884 hatte Sigmund FREUD (1856–1939), der allerdings andere therapeutische Erfolge damit suchte, die Aufmerksamkeit der Ärzte auf das Kokain gelenkt. Freud selbst berichtet darüber: „Im Juliheft des von Dr. HEITLER herausgegebenen Centralblattes für Therapie habe ich eine Studie über die Cocapflanze und deren Alkaloid Cocain veröffentlicht („Ueber Coca', Centralbl. f. d. ges. Therapie, vol. II, VII, July [not, as was frequently quoted: August] 1884), which brought this remedy to the attention of the doctors. A careful examination of the published reports and my own experiences showed this remedy to have been long-neglected. I may say that this suggestion brought an unexpectedly quick response. While Dr. KÖNIGSTEIN undertook at my request to test the analgesic and secretion-reducing properties of cocaine on the diseased conditions of the eye, Dr. Carl KOLLER, my colleague at the hospital, independently of my personal suggestion conceived the idea of producing a complete anaesthesia and analgesia of the cornea and conjunctiva by means of cocaine, whose anaesthetic effect on the sensibility of the mucous membrane had long been known (the seventh indication for the use of cocaine set up by me deals with the local application and ends with the words: 'Indeed, the anaesthetic properties of cocaine should make it suitable for a good many further applications'), and further demonstrated the immense practical value of this local anaesthetic through animal experimentations and operations on human beings. As a result of KOLLER's report on this matter to this year's Congress of Ophthalmologists at Heidelberg, cocaine has been generally accepted as a local anaesthetic."[95]

KOLLER, who wanted to become an ophthalmologist, had attended lectures on eye diseases held by Ferdinand von ARLT (1812–1887) during his medical studies. ARLT often complained in his lectures that in practice, general anaesthesia was unsuitable for use in ophthalmological surgery, not only because the assistance from the patient was highly desirable, but especially because of such side effects as nausea and vomiting. There was still no useful anaesthetic for eye surgery. KOLLER seriously wanted to find such a compound. It was natural that he should start experiments on local anaesthesia with such substances as chloral hydrate, bromides and morphine, though without any success. However, his first unsuccessful attempts made him receptive for recognizing a suitable anaesthetic immediately, should such a compound be found, unlike other researchers who overlooked it. KOLLER himself points to this fact in his "Supplemental Remarks on the Beginnings of Local Anaesthesia"[96] where he states: "The fact that cocaine makes lips and mucosa of the mouth and tongue 'numb' was noticed by everybody who came in touch with it. MORÉNO had even said in 1868 that this numbing effect might be of practical importance, and ANREP published

II. Jg., VII, Juli [nicht, wie vielfach fälschlich zitiert wurde: August] 1884), welche auf Grund einer Prüfung der in der Literatur enthaltenen Berichte und eigener Erfahrungen dieses lang vernachlässigte Mittel der Aufmerksamkeit der Aerzte empfahl. Ich darf sagen, dass der Erfolg dieser Anregung ein unerwartet rascher und vollkommener war. Während Herr Dr. L. Königstein auf mein Ersuchen es unternahm, die schmerzstillende und sekretioneinschränkende Wirksamkeit des Cocains in krankhaften Zuständen des Auges zu prüfen, hat mein Kollege in diesem Krankenhaus, Herr Dr. Karl Koller, unabhängig von meiner persönlichen Anregung, den glücklichen Gedanken gefasst, durch das Cocain, dessen abstumpfender Einfluss auf die Sensibilität der Schleimhäute seit langem bekannt ist (die siebente der von mir für den Gebrauch des Cocains aufgestellten Indikationen behandelt die örtliche Anwendung und schliesst mit den Worten: ‚Anwendungen, die auf der anästhesirenden Eigenschaft des Cocains beruhen, dürften sich wohl noch mehrere ergeben!'), eine vollständige Anästhesie und Analgesie der Cornea und Conjunctiva zu erzeugen, und hat fernerhin den hohen praktischen Werth dieser lokalen Anästhesie durch Thierversuche und Operationen am Menschen erwiesen. In Folge der darauf bezüglichen Mittheilung Koller's an den diesjährigen Kongress der Augenärzte zu Heidelberg ist das Cocain als lokales Anästetikum zur allgemeinen Aufnahme gelangt."[95]
Koller, der Augenarzt werden wollte, hatte schon in seiner Studienzeit bei Ferdinand von Arlt Vorlesungen über Augenkrankheiten gehört. Dabei hatte er eine besondere Schwierigkeit der operativen Ophthalmologie darin kennen gelernt, daß eine Allgemeinnarkose für dieses Fach kaum geeignet war. Deshalb nahm er sich ernstlich vor, ein Lokalanästhetikum für das Auge aufzufinden. Er suchte überall angespannt danach, in jedem nur irgendwie dazu geeigneten Medikament die Erfüllung seines Wunsches zu finden. So war er geeignet, ein etwa taugliches Anästhetikum, sollte es ihm nur irgendwie begegnen, sofort zu erkennen, und nicht wie andere Forscher einfach zu übersehen. Darauf verweist Koller in seinen „Nachträglichen Bemerkungen über die ersten Anfänge der Lokalanästhesie"[96], wo es weiter heißt: „Daß Kokain Lippen- und Zungenschleimhaut ‚taub' mache, war kaum jemandem entgangen, der es in Händen hatte. Ja, daß diese betäubende Wirkung einmal von praktischer Wichtigkeit werden könnte, hatte Moréno schon 1868 gesagt, und Anrep hatte dasselbe in einer ausgezeichneten, 1879 veröffentlichten physiologischen Arbeit ganz besonders hervorgehoben. Aber den tatsächlichen Versuch hatte vor mir niemand gemacht. Dazu war es nötig, daß das Kokain jemandem in die Hände fiel, der sich mit dem Gedanken einer zum Zwecke von Operationen erzeugten Lokalanästhesie trug. Nachdem ich mich von der Richtigkeit der Schlußfolgerung durch den Tierversuch und einige an mir selbst und an verschiedenen Kollegen gemachte Versuche überzeugt hatte, ließ ich am 15. September 1884 eine ‚Vorläufige Mitteilung' in der Sitzung der Deutschen Ophthalmologischen Gesellschaft zu Heidelberg verlesen und begleitende Experimente zeigen. . . . Jellinek [sic] wurde direkt von mir aufgefordert, das Kokain in Nase, Rachen und Kehlkopf zu verwenden. . . ."
Jelinek berichtete, wie bereits erwähnt, eine Woche später als ursprünglich angesetzt, also am 24. Oktober 1884, in der Gesellschaft der Ärzte über die „Anwendung des Cocains als Anästheticum und Analgeticum an der Schleimhaut des Rachens und Kehlkopfes"[97]. Jelinek berichtete ferner,[98] daß an excellent physiological study in 1879 in which he emphasized the same. But no one before me had tried the actual experiment. For this it was necessary that someone got his hands on cocaine who had been considering possibilities of a local anaesthesia for the purposes of operating. After I had convinced myself that my conclusions were correct by experimentation on animals and thereafter on myself and various colleagues, I had a preliminary communication read on September 15, 1884, at the German Society of Ophthalmologists in Heidelberg which was followed by a demonstration . . . Jellinek (sic) was asked by me to apply cocaine directly to the nose, pharynx and larynx . . ." As mentioned above, Jelinek reported to the Society of Physicians in Vienna on the use of "Cocaine as an Anaesthesia and Analgesia for the Mucous Membrane of the Pharynx and Larynx"[97] on October 24, 1884, a week later than originally planned. Moreover, Jelinek reported further[98] that Fauvel (Paris) found that pouring cocaine drop by drop into the larynx was a good method to make the vocal cords tense. But strangely enough practical applicability of the anaesthetizing effect went unmentioned. In his lecture Jelinek showed individual cases from Schrötter's clinic, for example, the removal of a laryngeal polyp under cocaine anaesthesia or a case of tuberculosis in which enormous relief for painful swallowing was attained. In an afterword Jelinek complained about the high cost of cocaine, however.

Of his own initiative Schrötter took up the new discovery and even published on the topic himself. Now that operations could be extended in length a whole new type of operative technique could be developed.

As previously mentioned Schrötter headed the laryngological clinic until 1890. For him, as a student of Skoda, the diseases of the thoracic cavity were of particular interest. When he became associate professor in 1875 he received the title as specialist for "throat and chest diseases". So for him the laryngological clinic was a building stone along the way to achieving a higher goal: the founding of a Third University Clinic of Medicine, which he eventually accomplished. But his real goal – that of uniting the existing Clinic of Laryngology with the new clinic of internal medicine under his leadership – remained unfulfilled. The College of Professors and the Administration could only decide against setting a precedent by unifying two clinics of two different disciplines under one head, so Schrötter was forced to choose between them: he chose to lead the Clinic of Internal Medicine.

Schrötter, whose great interest concerned diseases of the thoracic cavity as already stated, succeeded in establishing the first Public Sanatorium for Tuberculosis in Austria (Alland) shortly before the turn of the century and only after great difficulties. He sent his student Josef Sorgo (1869–1950) there, whom he had trained at his Third University Clinic of Medicine seven years previously. Sorgo introduced treatment of the inner larynx using sunlight,[99] which was to have an influence later on the treatment of extrapulmonary tuberculosis by sunlight.[100]

Schrötter had hundreds of pupils all over the world. Among his close co-workers who were either his assistants or secondary physicians the following should be mentioned: Georg Catti, Georg Juffinger, Eduard Ronsburger (1838–1905), Ottokar Chiari, and Geza Georg Kobler (1864–1935). Hermann Arthur Thost (1854–1937) founded the University Clinic of Oto-Laryngology in Hamburg.

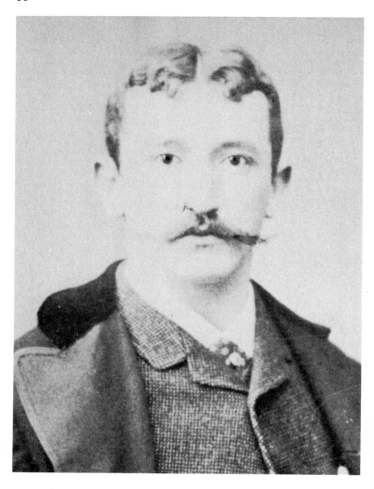

Karl Koller. Photographie aus dem Jahr 1883.
Koller entdeckte die anästhesierende Fähigkeit einer wäßrigen Lösung von Cocainum muriaticum im Institut für allgemeine und experimentelle Pathologie und erprobte die Wirkung dieses Lokalanästhetikums an der II. Universitäts-Augenklinik.

Karl Koller. Photograph, 1883.
Koller discovered the anaesthetizing property of a watery solution of Cocainum muriaticum at the Institute of General and Experimental Pathology. He tested the effects of this local anaesthesia at the Second University Clinic of Ophthalmology.

ÜBER COCA.

Von

DR. SIGM. FREUD

Secundararzt im k. k. Allgemeinen Krankenhause
in Wien.

Neu durchgesehener und vermehrter Separat-Abdruck aus dem
„Centralblatt für die gesammte Therapie".

WIEN, 1885.
VERLAG VON MORITZ PERLES
Stadt, Bauernmarkt Nr. 11.

Mit seiner Arbeit „Über Coca" lenkte Sigmund Freud im Jahr 1884 die Aufmerksamkeit der Ärzte auf das Kokain. Abgebildet ist das Titelblatt des „neu durchgesehenen und vermehrten Separat-Abdrucks aus dem ‚Centralblatt für die gesammte Therapie'", Wien 1885. Dort schreibt Freud am Ende der „Nachträge": „Zur localen Wirkung des Cocains. Diese Indication für den Cocagebrauch ist durch die Anwendung von Koller zur Anästhesirung der Hornhaut, durch die Arbeiten von Königstein, Jelinek und ungezählten anderen zur allgemeinsten Anerkennung gelangt und sichert dem Cocain einen bleibenden Werth im Arzneischatze."

Edmund Jelinek. Nach einer zeitgenössischen Originalphotographie. Jelinek berichtete am 24. Oktober 1884 in der Gesellschaft der Ärzte in Wien über die „Anwendung des Cocains als Anästheticum und Analgeticum an der Schleimhaut des Rachens und Kehlkopfes". In seinem Vortrag zeigte Jelinek auch bereits einzelne Fälle aus der Klinik Schrötter, so die Entfernung eines Kehlkopfpolypen in Kokainanästhesie und einen Fall von Tuberkulose, wobei eine außerordentliche Erleichterung des schmerzhaften Schluckaktes erreicht wurde. Dadurch brach eine neue Ära in der Laryngologie an.

Edmund Jelinek. Contemporary photograph.
On October 24, 1884, Jelinek reported to the Society of Physicians in Vienna on the use of "Cocaine as an Anaesthesia and Analgesia for the Mucous Membrane of the Pharynx and Larynx". In his lecture Jelinek showed individual cases from Schrötter's clinic, for example, the removal of a laryngeal polyp under cocaine anaesthesia or a case of tuberculosis in which enormous relief for painful swallowing was attained. A new era in laryngology had begun.

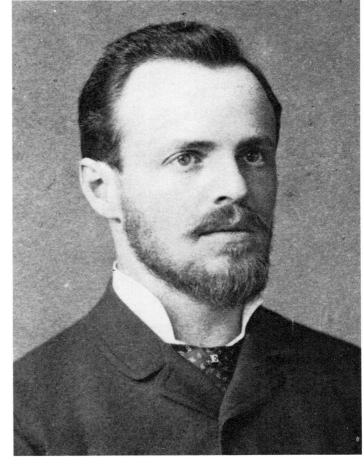

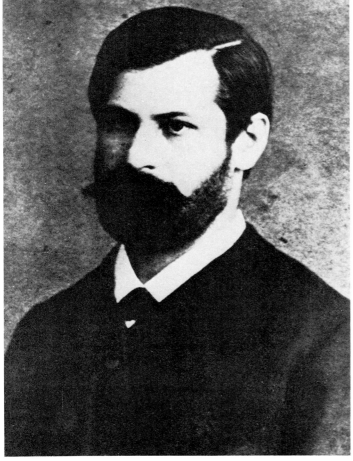

In 1884 Sigmund Freud called his colleagues' attention to cocaine with his work "Über Coca". Pictured is the title page to the "newly revised and reprinted separate edition from the 'Centralblatt für die gesammte Therapie'", Vienna, 1885. Freud closes with the words: "On the local effects of cocaine. This indication for the use of cocaine received general recognition through Koller's anaesthetizing of the cornea, through the works of Königstein, Jelinek and numerous others and guarantees cocaine a lasting medicinal value."

im Einträufeln von Kokain am Kehlkopf FAUVEL in Paris ein gutes Spannungsmittel der Stimmbänder gefunden habe. Die praktische Verwertbarkeit aber der anäesthesierenden Wirkung blieb merkwürdigerweise aus. In seinem Vortrag zeigte JELINEK auch bereits einzelne Fälle aus der Klinik SCHRÖTTER, so die Entfernung eines Kehlkopfpolypen in Kokainanästhesie und einen Fall von Tuberkulose, wobei eine außerordentliche Erleichterung des schmerzhaften Schluckaktes erreicht wurde. In einem Nachtrag beklagt JELINEK allerdings auch den hohen Preis des Cocains.

Mit der ihm eigenen Energie griff SCHRÖTTER die neue Entdeckung auf, ja er publizierte sogar selbst darüber. Jetzt konnte die operative Technik erst richtig entwickelt werden, war es doch nunmehr möglich, Operationen in beliebiger zeitlicher Ausdehnung durchzuführen.

Wie schon erwähnt, leitete SCHRÖTTER die laryngologische Klinik bis zum Jahr 1890. Für ihn, den SKODA-Schüler, stellten die Krankheiten des Brustraumes ein besonderes Anliegen dar, und als er 1875 zum außerordentlichen Professor ernannt wurde, erhielt er diesen Titel mit dem Prädikat „für Hals- und Brustkrankheiten". So war für ihn die laryngologische Klinik letztlich ein Baustein auf dem Weg zur Erreichung eines höheren Zieles: der Gründung und Errichtung einer III. Medizinischen Universitätsklinik, was ihm schließlich auch gelang. Aber sein eigentliches Ziel, die Vereinigung der schon bestehenden laryngologischen Klinik mit der neuen internen Klinik in seiner Hand, blieb ihm versagt: Professorenkollegium und Unterrichtsverwaltung konnten sich zur Statuierung eines Exempels, der Vereinigung zweier Kliniken verschiedenen Faches unter einem Vorstand, nicht entschließen, und so sah sich SCHRÖTTER vor die Wahl gestellt, sich für eine von den beiden zu entscheiden: er wählte die interne Klinik.

SCHRÖTTER, dem wie schon gesagt, die Krankheiten des Brustraumes ein besonderes Anliegen waren, gelang es noch knapp vor der Jahrhundertwende, nach langwierigen Auseinandersetzungen, die erste Volksheilstätte für Tuberkulosekranke in Österreich (Alland) zu schaffen. Dorthin sandte er 1902 seinen Schüler Josef SORGO (1869–1950), den er sieben Jahre vorher an seiner, der III. Medizinischen Klinik, ausgebildet hatte. SORGO führte die Sonnenlichtbehandlung des Kehlkopfinneren[99] ein, die einen großen Einfluß auf die Sonnenlichtbehandlung der extrapulmonalen Tuberkulose gewann.[100]

Von SCHRÖTTERS engeren Schülern sind insbesondere Georg CATTI, Georg JUFFINGER, Eduard RONSBURGER (1838–1905), Ottokar CHIARI und Geza Georg KOBLER (1864–1935) zu nennen. Hermann Arthur THOST (1854–1937) begründete die Hamburger Universitätsklinik für Oto-Laryngologie. SCHRÖTTERS Sohn Hermann VON SCHRÖTTER (1870–1928) „arbeitete auch viel auf der Klinik seines Vaters und war ein geschickter Laryngoskopiker", schreibt Thost.[101] „Er hatte eine sehr geschickte, glückliche Hand, und als man über den Kehlkopf hinaus tief in die Lunge und die Bronchien eindrang, war er einer der ersten, der diese Kunst mit ausbildete und verbesserte. Sein Buch über Bronchoskopie [erschienen 1906] war eines der besten, das damals erschien. Alles Technische beherrschte er, war nicht nur Arzt, sondern auch Ingenieur."

Nachfolger SCHRÖTTERS als Vorstand der laryngologischen Klinik wurde 1891 der ehemalige Sekundararzt TÜRCKS, Carl STOERK. Er führte als unbesoldeter Extraordinarius die Klinik SCHRÖTTER's son, Hermann VON SCHRÖTTER (1870–1928) "worked in his father's department and was a skilled laryngoscopist", according to THOST.[101] "He concentrated on the clinical use of bronchoscopy, on which subject he wrote his much-quoted monograph of the same title in 1906. He was technically well-versed and was not only a physician but also an engineer."

In 1891 SCHRÖTTER was succeeded as head of the laryngological clinic by TÜRCK's former chief assistant, Carl STOERK. STOERK remained in this post until his death in 1899, but this was an unpaid appointment as associate professor. While SCHRÖTTER in 1890 received a paid appointment from the government, when he became full professor and head of the Third Medical Clinic, "STOERK never reached this goal; . . . Only the third head of the Department of Laryngology, Ottokar CHIARI, succeeded in winning two important points at the start of the 20th century: the recognition of rhinolaryngology as a compulsory subject of study in the curriculum of 1903 regulating the study of medicine; and two years later the elevation of the chair to a salaried associate professorship integrated in the medical curriculum."[102]

Carl STOERK, born in Ofen (Hungary) in 1832, graduated in Vienna in 1858, and in 1864 applied for the position as lecturer in "laryngo- and rhinoscopy and diseases of the larynx, the trachea and the pharynx", and was "the first and only one to dedicate all his time to this specialty."[103] This statement is correct in as far as "STOERK's friend and co-worker in laryngological research, Friedrich SEMELEDER (1832–1901), born in Wiener Neustadt, was also appointed lecturer in laryngology and rhinology in 1861, but he had worked as a consulting physician in the surgical department of the Gumpendorf hospital, and when STOERK made the above statement in 1869 he had been abroad for five years. His Mexican adventure as personal physician to Maximilian von Hapsburg was already behind him, but in contrast to his colleague Samuel von BASCH (1837–1905) he had not returned to his homeland but had settled in Cordoba, Mexico, where he died in 1901, greatly honored as the founder of the Academia Nacional de Medicina de México."[104] SEMELEDER, together with TÜRCK, CZERMAK and STOERK, belongs to the men who in Austria in 1858 "stood at the cradle of laryngology."[105]

SEMELEDER, encouraged by his teacher CZERMAK, was especially interested in rhinoscopy. "In 1862 SEMELEDER published the monograph 'Die Rhinoskopie und ihr Werth für die ärztliche Praxis' (Eng. ed. 'Rhinoscopy and Laryngoscopy: Their Value in Practical Medicine.' 1886) (Leipzig, 1862), in which he formulated the doctrine of giving 'this new examination method its rightful appreciation.' With this plan, the examiner needed to have both hands free, which CZERMAK also felt when he advised holding the mirror in the mouth by means of a handle. It proved more convenient, however, to wear the mirror fixed to a pair of glasses. Such an instrument, devised by SEMELEDER, was one of the stops on the road to the forehead reflector which TÜRCK eventually introduced in laryngological practice. SEMELEDER was rather happy that even the otologists Ignaz GRUBER and Adam POLITZER adopted his spectacle-mirror. Just as he worked in close cooperation with those two, especially with POLITZER, in refining the technique of tube catheterization, SEMELEDER also kept very close contact with STOERK, who at that time was secondary physician at TÜRCK's department."[106]

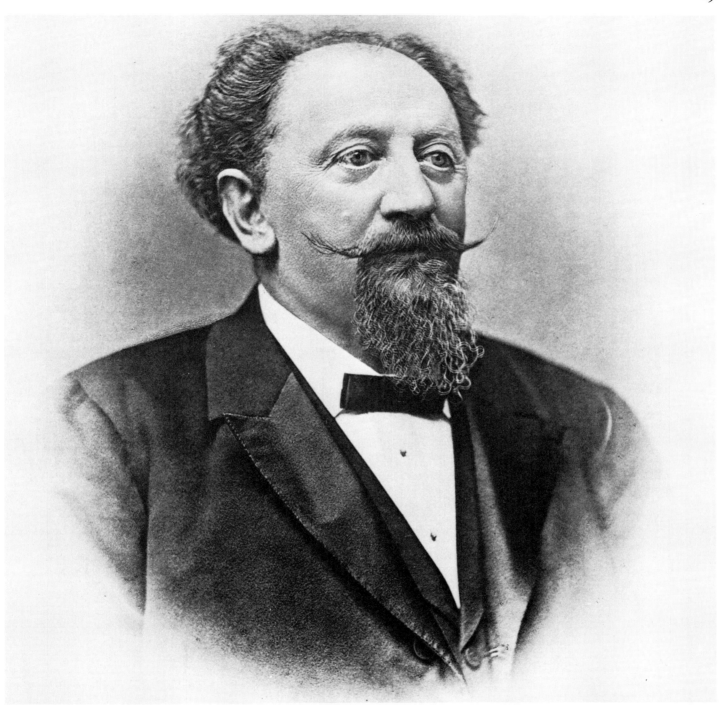

Karl Stoerk.
Nach einem Lichtdruck von J. Löwy, Wien.

Karl Stoerk.
Heliograph by J. Löwy, Vienna.

bis zu seinem Tod 1899. Während SCHRÖTTER durch seine Ernennung zum Ordinarius der III. Medizinischen Klinik eine besoldete staatliche Anstellung erlangte, hat „STOERK sie zeit seines Lebens nicht erlangt. Denn als er ... die Leitung der laryngologischen Klinik übernahm ... tat er dies in der Eigenschaft eines unbesoldeten Extraordinarius. Erst dem dritten laryngologischen Klinikchef, Ottokar CHIARI, ist am Anfang des 20. Jahrhunderts beides gelungen: die Anerkennung der Laryngo-Rhinologie als obligates Lehrfach in der Studienordnung von 1903. Zwei Jahre später folgte 1905 auch die Erhebung der Lehrkanzel zu einem systemisierten Extraordinariat."[102]

Der 1832 in Ofen geborene STOERK wurde 1858 in Wien promoviert und habilitierte sich 1864 für Laryngo- und Rhinoskopie und Krankheiten des Kehlkopfes, der Luftröhre und des Rachens und war „der erste Privatdocent für diese Fächer"[103]. Dies ist insofern richtig, weil „STOERKS Freund und laryngologischer Mitforscher, der in Wiener Neustadt geborene Friedrich SEMELEDER (1832–1901), ... sich schon 1861 ebenfalls für Laryngo- und Rhinoskopie habilitiert hatte, aber als ordinierender Arzt an der chirurgischen Abteilung des Gumpendorfer Spitals tätig gewesen (war) und 1869, als Stoerk diese Feststellung machte, fünf Jahre außer Landes (weilte)." Er hatte nämlich als Leibarzt Maximilian von Habsburg nach Mexiko begleitet und sich später in Cordoba niedergelassen, wo er „in großen Ehren als Begründer der Academia Nacional de Medicina de México 1901"[104] starb; er gehört – mit TÜRCK, CZERMAK und STOERK – zu jenen Männern, die in Österreich 1858 „an der Wiege der Laryngologie"[105] standen.

SEMELEDER widmete sich, angeregt durch seinen Lehrer CZERMAK, besonders der Rhinoskopie. „Mit seiner 1862 erschienenen Monographie ‚Die Rhinoskopie und ihr Werth für die ärztliche Praxis' (Leipzig 1862) will SEMELEDER programmatisch ‚dieser neuen Untersuchungsweise zu jener Geltung verhelfen, die ihr gebührt.' Bei ihr besonders mußte man beide Hände zum Hantieren frei haben. Diese Notwendigkeit hat auch CZERMAK gefühlt, als er empfahl, den Spiegel mittels eines Stieles im Munde zu fixieren. Da war es doch zweckmäßiger, ihn in Verbindung mit einer Brille zutragen. SEMELEDERS Brillenspiegel stellt nur eine der Stationen dar auf dem Wege zum Stirnreflektor, den TÜRCK endgültig in die laryngologische Praxis einführte. Es war für SEMELEDER keine geringe Freude, daß sogar die Ohrenärzte, Ignaz GRUBER und Adam POLITZER, seinen Brillenspiegel adoptierten. Wie SEMELEDER mit diesen beiden, vor allem mit POLITZER, beim Ausbau des Tubenkatheterismus zusammenarbeitete, so stand er auch im engsten Kontakt mit dem damaligen Sekundarius TÜRCKS, mit STOERK."[106]

STOERKS Hauptinteresse galt dem Kehlkopf. So war er nach seinen eigenen Angaben der erste, der unter Verwendung des TÜRCKschen Kehlkopfspiegels Medikamente in den Kehlkopf einbrachte. Schon 1859 erteilte er in Privatkursen im Allgemeinen Krankenhaus Unterricht in der Laryngoskopie, und zwar zunächst an der Leiche. Auch an Tieren stellte STOERK schon damals Untersuchungen an, ja er mietete sich sogar einen eigenen Tierstall in Ottakring, einerseits um sich in Übung beim Laryngoskopieren zu halten, andererseits um die Kehlkopfbewegungen zu studieren. Auch an sich selbst „experimentierte" er, um die damals drängenden Fragen nach der zweckmäßigsten Beleuchtungs- und Spiegeltechnik zu erforschen. SEMELEDER führte sich eine Schlundzange in die

The main interest of STOERK was the larynx. He worked out numerous technical details for examining this organ and he also claimed for himself to have been the first one who, by means of TÜRCK's laryngeal mirror, applied medications to the larynx for therapeutical purposes. As early as 1859 he held private courses in laryngoscopy, first using cadavers in the Vienna General Hospital and later animals. He even rented an animal stable in Vienna's district of Ottakring in order to practice laryngoscopy on animals and to study the movements of the larynx. STOERK also carried out experiments on himself in order to study the still unsolved problems of finding the most efficient techniques of illuminating and mirroring. SEMELEDER did the same: he, for instance, introduced a pharyngeal forceps into his esophagus, and his friend "STOERK could look a little deeper than is usually possible with the aid of the mirror." This new method was then practiced on a patient with a disease of the esophagus: "It was possible to see to just below the lower border of the cricoid cartilage, i. e., more than an inch into the esophagus, but more was not possible in this case."[107] However primitive the attempts of SEMELEDER and STOERK may have been in the winter of 1861–62, they nevertheless represent the beginning of esophagoscopy. STOERK's attempts to improve illumination led him to use the already mentioned "Schusterkugel", a glass ball filled with water to collect the light. "However, all this appears to be of little value when compared with the daring venture of not only looking into the larynx but also performing operations inside this organ. STOERK could justly claim to have been the first to do so. With an especially constructed lapis-holder he cauterized the ulcerated mucosa of the larynx in a case of laryngeal syphilis; spasm of the glottis, a dreaded complication of the prelaryngoscopic era, did not occur. The time had now arrived for local therapy of the larynx. In view of the treatment methods which came into use, painting, cauterizing, incising and inhalating, it is in the larynx that this method has been of the greatest benefit. A veritable arsenal of laryngeal instruments evolved: holders for cauterizing substances, blowers for powders, laryngeal forceps, brushes, syringes, covered and uncovered laryngeal scalpels and guillotines, scissors and tourniquets. STOERK showed unlimited ingenuity in the construction of new instruments. By 1869, their inventor could boast in a letter to the ministry of thirty inventions, and he also pointed out that through him 'Vienna has become the main production center of laryngological instruments'".[108] And STOERK also knew how to use these instruments with incomparable virtuosity. He had the reputation of being the most skilled endolaryngeal surgeon before the discovery of cocaine. In 1862 he had been the second to successfully remove a laryngeal polyp. (Viktor VON BRUNS in Tübingen did this for the first time in 1861.) As previously mentioned, STOERK, due to his thorough training in surgery, was excellently qualified for such operations and "this surgical schooling of the Viennese laryngologists should certainly not be forgotten, despite their basically internistic origin."[109]

In his scientific publications STOERK dealt with nearly all the important questions of laryngoscopy. As early as 1899, however, most of his methods and the instruments which he described in his books were already outdated. "Besides, one of STOERK's most eminent works, 'Chronic Blennorrhea of the Mucous Membranes of the Nose, Larynx and Trachea', is only of historical interest nowadays, since this pathological

Speiseröhre ein, und Freund „STOERK vermochte mit dem Spiegel etwas tiefer hinabzusehen als es gewöhnlich gelingt" und im Anschluß daran praktizierten die beiden das Verfahren bei einem Speiseröhrenkranken: „Man konnte bis unter den unteren Ringknorpelrand, sohin mehr als einen Zoll tief in die Speiseröhre sehen und um mehr handelte es sich in diesem Falle nicht."[107] Diese Bemühungen von STOERK und SEMELEDER im Winter 1861/62 mit einem Spiegel in den oberen Anteil der Speiseröhre zu blicken, stellen, auch wenn sie primitiv waren, die Anfänge der Ösophagoskopie dar. Seine Bemühungen, die Beleuchtung zu verbessern, führte ihn, wie schon früher erwähnt, zur Anwendung der Schusterkugel, einer mit Wasser gefüllten Glaskugel, zur Sammlung des Lichtes. „Was aber wog dies alles gegenüber dem kühnen Unterfangen, nicht nur in den Kehlkopf hineinzuschauen, sondern auch in ihn hineinzugreifen. STOERK darf sich rühmen, es als erster getan zu haben. Mit einem eigens konstruierten Lapisträger ätzte er erstmals bei einem Fall von Kehlkopflues die geschwürig veränderte Kehlkopfschleimhaut. Der in der vorlaryngoskopischen Ära so sehr gefürchtete Glottiskrampf trat nicht ein. Die Stunde der Lokaltherapie war nunmehr für den Kehlkopf gekommen. Mit den Methoden des Pinselns, Ätzens, Schneidens und Inhalierens hat sie gerade an diesem Organ ihre größten Erfolge erzielt. Ein wahres Arsenal von Kehlkopfinstrumenten, von Ätzmittelträgern, Pulverbläsern, Kehlkopfpinzetten, Pinseln, Spritzen, gedeckten und ungedeckten Larynxmessern und Guillotinen, Scheren und Quetschschlingen entstand. STOERK war schier unerschöpflich in der Erfindung immer neuer Instrumente. 1869 sind es bereits 30, als deren Erfinder er sich vor dem Ministerium rühmen und zugleich darauf hinweisen kann, daß so durch ihn ‚Wien der Hauptbezugsplatz für laryngologische Instrumente' weithin geworden ist."[108] Und STOERK wußte diese Instrumente mit einer Virtuosität ohnegleichen auch anzuwenden, so daß er mit Recht als der gewandteste endolaryngeale Operateur vor der Entdeckung des Kokains galt, war es doch STOERK 1862 als zweitem gelungen, einen Kehlkopfpolypen abzutragen. (Vor ihm hatte 1861 Viktor VON BRUNS in Tübingen einen derartigen Eingriff erfolgreich ausgeführt.) Wie schon früher darauf hingewiesen, brachte STOERK auf Grund seiner chirurgischen Ausbildung bei Franz SCHUH dafür beste Voraussetzungen mit und man darf „diese chirurgische Schulung gerade der Wiener Laryngologen ... nicht vergessen, auch wenn ihre internistische Herkunft im Vordergrund steht."[109]

In seinen wissenschaftlichen Publikationen beschäftigte sich STOERK mit beinahe allen wichtigen Fragen der Laryngoskopie; allerdings wurde bereits 1899 an ihnen kritisiert, daß viele der von STOERK angegebenen Methoden und Instrumente bereits der Geschichte angehörten. „Ebenso besitzt eine der bedeutendsten Arbeiten STOERK's: ‚Die chronische Blennorrhoe der Nasen-, Kehlkopf- und Luftröhren-Schleimhaut' gegenwärtig nur mehr ein geschichtliches Interesse, da ja diese Krankheitsform, wenn auch nicht vollkommen, so doch zum grössten Theile als zum Rhinosklerom gehörig angesehen wird. Immerhin hat sich STOERK durch die Erkenntnis dieser merkwürdigen Krankheit ein grosses, unvergängliches Verdienst erworben."[110] Erna LESKY verweist darauf, daß es kein Zufall war, weshalb sich viele Wiener Kliniker seit den siebziger Jahren des vorigen Jahrhunderts mit dem Rhinosklerom beschäftigten. Damals bildete der ganze Südosten Europas das Einzugsgebiet für die Patienten des Allgemeinen Kranken-

phenomenon is now regarded as belonging for the most part to rhinoscleroma. STOERK, however, has won for himself great and everlasting merits by observing and studying this strange disease."[110] Erna LESKY explains why so many of the Viennese clinicians since the 1870s were interested in rhinoscleroma: "At that time the whole southeastern part of Europa was the hinterland, as it were, which supplied patients to the General Hospital. And from this part of Europe, from Moravia, Galicia, Poland, Walachia, and Bessarabia, came the cases in whom STOERK, by means of his laryngoscope, found the same granulations in the larynx and trachea, which had already been described in the nose and mouth as rhinoscleroma by the dermatologists ... All this work was summarized in 1892 by STOERK's assistant of that period, the later laryngologist of Innsbruck, Georg JUFFINGER (1853–1913), in the monograph 'Scleroma of the Mucosae of the Nose, the Pharynx, the Larynx and the Trachea' (Leipzig and Vienna, 1892). No wonder that STOERK, who had done research on this disease his whole life, expanded the chapters on blennorrhea and rhinoscleroma in his textbooks to become rather detailed monographs with many case reports and statistical data."[111]

In addition to the laryngological clinic in the Vienna General Hospital there was another place in Vienna where, from 1872, laryngology was taught and studied; i. e., the Department of Laryngology of the General Policlinic. The department was headed by Johann SCHNITZLER (1835–1893; M. D. 1860, lecturer 1865, "titular" associate professor 1878, director of the General Policlinic 1884) from 1872 until his death in 1893. SCHNITZLER like all other prominent laryngologists of that period was originally an internal specialist, and practiced internal medicine throughout his life. The attempts of the founders of the Policlinic to create an institution where all branches of medicine should be practiced by specialists led to a separation of the fields of work. SCHNITZLER, who had already shown interest in the still young specialty and who had already published scientific papers on the subject, began to treat diseases of the throat and the thoracic organs and also lectured on them. To these were added lectures on laryngoscopy and rhinoscopy combined with practical instructions as well as clinical lectures on diseases of the larynx, the pharynx and the nose. In 1878, SCHNITZLER could already point to the fact "that in the six years of his activity in the Policlinic, no less than 500 students had attended his courses, of whom 175 came from Germany, 118 from the United States, 62 from Russia, and even 10 young physicians from Asia and 2 from Australia had come to study under him."[112] SCHNITZLER was open to all new methods in his specialty, and he was among the first to use inhalation therapy after its introduction in 1862. In the mid-eighties he was the first in Vienna to use hypnosis in treating laryngeal diseases. His son and assistant of that period Arthur SCHNITZLER (1862–1931) later used such an experiment, the treatment of a twenty-year-old girl by means of hypnosis who had been suffering for a number of weeks from aphonia and choking attacks, as material for his one-act play "Paracelsus". In compliance with the then current psychoanalytical research – in 1893 Sigmund FREUD and Josef BREUER published together as a preliminary communication their observations "On the Psychological Mechanism of Hysterical Phenomena" and in 1895 their "Studies on Hysteria" appeared – Arthur SCHNITZLER treated the hysterical symptoms of his patient in the play by means of catharsis.

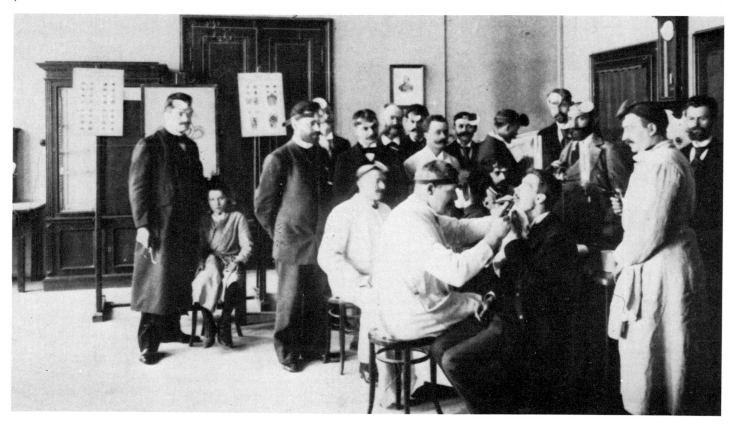

| D. Der ärztliche Dienst in der Poliklinik während des Jahres 1872. ||||
Tägliche Ordinationen (Sonn- und Feiertage ausgenommen)	Tages-Zeit. Uhr	Ordinirende Aerzte	Assistenten	Aspiranten
Für innere Krankheiten, besonders Lungen- u. Herzkrankheiten, von October b. Mai	1—2	Docent Dr. Rollett.	Dr. Emanuel Kramer. Dr. Ignaz Lindner.	— —
Für innere Krankheiten, besonders der Hals- und Brustorgane	8—9	Docent Dr. Schnitzler.	Dr. Raffaello Coen.	Dr. Julius Sterk.
Für innere Krankheiten, besonders der Bauchorgane	5—6	Primararzt Dr. Oser.	Dr. Josef Löbl. Dr. Ignaz Fränkl.	— —
Für innere Krankheiten, besonders Nervenkrankheiten mit Elektrotherapie	8—9	Professor Dr. Schwanda.	Dr. Emerich Klotzberg.	— —
Für innere Krankheiten, besond. Gemüths- u. Nervenkr., Montag, Mittwoch u. Freitag	1—2	Prof. Dr. Leidesdorf.	Dr. Leopold Weinberger	— —
Für innere Krankheiten, (Hydrotherapie).	10—11	Docent Dr. Winternitz.	Dr. Sigismund Baum.	Dr. R. Suter, Dr. H. Wollensack, N. Wolfenstein.
Für chirurgische Krankheiten	3—4	Docent Dr. Neudörfer.	Dr. Carl Egger, k.k.O.-A.	Dr. Emil Amrusch und Drd. Josef Minigerode.
Für chirurgische Krankheiten, besonders der Harnorgane	11—12	Docent Dr. Ultzmann.	Dr. Julius Beregszászy Dr. Leopold Weinberger	Drd. Richard v.d. Hoope.
Für Hautkrankheiten und Syphilis	12—1	Primararzt Dr. Auspitz.	Dr. Benno Berger.	Drd. Adolf Stern.
Für Augenkrankheiten	½10—11	Docent Dr. Hock.	Dr. Maxim. Munk.	Drd. Jacob Munk.
Für Augenkrankheiten	1—2	Docent Dr. v. Reuss.	Dr. Adolf Schlesinger.	— —
Für Ohrenkrankheiten	4—5	Dr. Urbantschitsch.	— —	Drd Leopold Nied.
Für Kinderkrankheiten	3—4	Docent Dr. Fleischmann	— —	Drd. Ed. Suchatzky.
Für Kinderkrankheiten	10—11	Docent Dr. Monti.	— —	Drd. Adolf Jarisch.
Für Frauenkrankheiten	11—12	Doc. Dr. Carl Rokitansky.	Dr. Baptist Sauer.	Drd. Felix Ehrendorfer.

Oben: Laryngologische Ambulanz der Wiener Poliklinik.
Unten: Im Jahr 1872 behandelte Johann Schnitzler an der Poliklinik „innere Krankheiten, besonders der Hals- und Brustorgane" und Viktor von Urbantschitsch „Ohrenkrankheiten".
Aus: Jahresbericht der allgemeinen Poliklinik in Wien für 1872. Wien 1873.

Top: Laryngological out-patient department of the Vienna General Policlinic.
Bottom: In 1872 Johann Schnitzler treated "internal diseases, especially those of the throat and thorax" and Viktor von Urbantschitsch treated "diseases of the ear" in the Vienna General Policlinic.

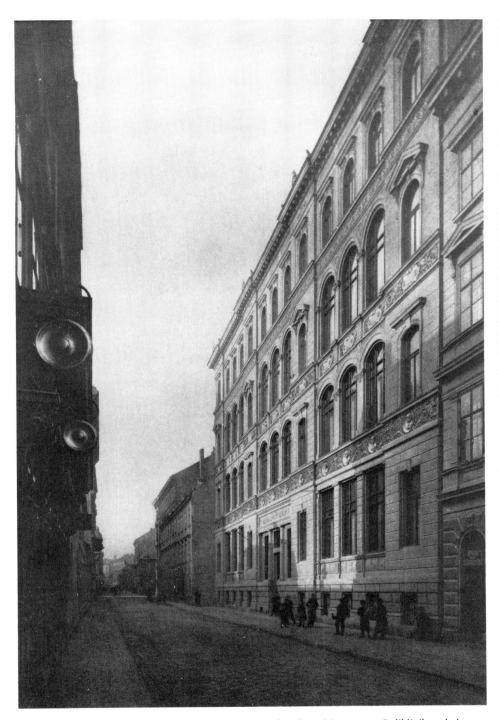
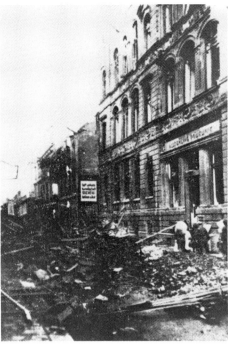
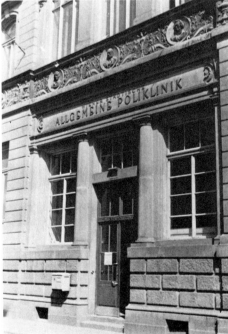

Vorderfront der Wiener Allgemeinen Poliklinik um 1900.

Front view of the Vienna General Policlinic around 1900.

Rechts oben: Die zerstörte Poliklinik nach der Bombardierung vom 4. 11. 1944.

Top right: The Policlinic after the bombardment of November 4, 1944.

Rechts unten: Eingang zur Poliklinik nach der Restaurierung.

Bottom right: Entrance to the Policlinic after its restoration.

hauses und aus diesem Südosten Europas stammten die Fälle, an denen STOERK mit seinem Laryngoskop dieselben Granulationen an Kehlkopf und Trachea beobachtete, die die Dermatologen an Nase und Mund bereits als Rhinosklerom beschrieben hatten. Ottokar CHIARI und Gustav RIEHL haben in der Klinik SCHRÖTTER die Symptomatologie und den Verlauf der Krankheit geklärt. „Ihre zusammenfassende Darstellung hat sie 1892 in der Monographie des damaligen STOERK-Assistenten und späteren Innsbrucker Laryngologen Georg JUFFINGER (1853–1913) ‚Sklerom der Schleimhaut der Nase, des Rachens, des Kehlkopfes und der Luftröhre' (Leipzig und Wien 1892) erfahren. Kein Wunder, daß der Forscher, der sich ein Leben lang mit diesem Krankheitsbild beschäftigte, STOERK, die Blennorrhoe bzw. Rhinosklerom-Kapitel seiner Lehrbücher zu detailreichen Monographien mit reicher Kasuistik und Statistik auswachsen ließ."[111]

Seit 1872 gab es neben der laryngologischen Klinik im Allgemeinen Krankenhaus noch eine andere laryngologische Lehr- und Lernstätte in Wien, nämlich die laryngologische Abteilung der Allgemeinen Poliklinik, die von Johann SCHNITZLER (1835–1893; Dr. med. 1860, Doz. 1865, Titularextraordinarius 1878, Direktor der Allgemeinen Poliklinik ab 1884) von 1872 bis zu seinem Tod 1893 geleitet wurde. SCHNITZLER kam, so wie damals alle anderen prominenten Laryngologen, von der internen Medizin und führte auch zeit seines Lebens die allgemeine internistische Praxis fort. Das Bemühen der Gründer der Poliklinik, diese zu einem Institut zu machen, das für alle Teilgebiete der praktischen Medizin, dem damaligen Stand ihrer Entwicklung entsprechend, offen war, führte zu einer Teilung der Arbeitsgebiete. SCHNITZLER, der sich bereits vielfach mit der noch jungen Laryngologie beschäftigt und auch bereits eine Reihe von Arbeiten darüber veröffentlicht hatte, übernahm die Erkrankungen der Hals- und Brustorgane und auch seine Vorlesungen trugen diesen Titel. Hinzu kamen Vorlesungen über Laryngoskopie und Rhinoskopie mit praktischen Übungen, sodann klinische Vorlesungen über die Krankheiten des Kehlkopfs, Rachens und der Nase. Im Jahr 1878 konnte Johann SCHNITZLER bereits darauf hinweisen, daß er in den sechs Jahren seiner Tätigkeit an der Poliklinik 500 Hörer gehabt hatte, davon 175 aus Deutschland, 118 aus den Vereinigten Staaten, 62 aus Rußland; ja selbst Asien und Australien waren mit 10 bzw. 2 Hörern vertreten.[112] Als einer der ersten führte SCHNITZLER schon 1862 die Inhalationstherapie ein. Zur Behandlung von Kehlkopfneurosen verwendete SCHNITZLER auch die Hypnose. Sein Sohn und damaliger Assistent Arthur SCHNITZLER (1862–1931) verwertete literarisch die Heilung einer hysterischen Aphonie in seinem Einakter ‚Paracelsus'. Ganz in Übereinstimmung mit der damals aktuellen psychoanalytischen Forschung – 1893 veröffentlichten Sigmund FREUD und Josef BREUER ihre Erfahrungen über eine neue Methode der Erforschung und Behandlung hysterischer Phänomene in einer „Vorläufigen Mitteilung" und 1895 erschienen ihre „Studien über Hysterie" – läßt Arthur SCHNITZLER die Hysterikerin durch „Abreagieren", durch Bewußtmachen uneingestandener, verborgener Regungen gesund werden. Am 19. März 1898 urteilte FREUD über SCHNITZLERS ‚Paracelsus': „Unlängst war ich in SCHNITZLERS ‚Paracelsus' erstaunt, wieviel von den Dingen so ein Dichter weiß."[113] Dies ist freilich gar nicht so verwunderlich, verfaßte SCHNITZLER doch sogar eine wissenschaftliche Arbeit darüber: „Über funktionelle Aphonie und deren Behandlung durch Hypnose und Sugge-

"Recently I attended a performance of SCHNITZLER's 'Paracelsus' and I was surprised how much a playwright knows about these matters', FREUD stated in 1898.[113] This does not come as a surprise, however, since Arthur SCHNITZLER published a scientific work on research done on this subject entitled "On Functional Aphonia and Its Treatment by Means of Hypnosis and Suggestion".[114] More than once the writer-physician Arthur SCHNITZLER created a sensation, as for instance when in 1913 his comedy in five acts "Professor Bernhardi" was forbidden on the stage "in order to safeguard public interests". Its first performance in Vienna took place in 1920, but even in 1946 it was argued whether the play should be performed on the stage or not.[115] The plot consists of an affair which is wholly fictional, but is closely connected to Johann SCHNITZLER's position as founding member of the Policlinic and its director, and the hostilities and envy he had to face.

The tuberculosis problem had also engaged Johann SCHNITZLER's interest, and when Robert KOCH in 1890 published his new treatment methods, SCHNITZLER in the autumn of the same year performed a series of experiments in his department with KOCH's remedy.[116]

In 1892 Johann SCHNITZLER had been able to experience the joy of moving the Policlinic to the new, and for that time, ultra-progressively equipped building in Mariannengasse. The department which he shared with URBANTSCHITSCH consisted of a waiting-room, two consulting rooms and a lecture room on the first floor.

After Johann SCHNITZLER's death the primarii of the Policlinic's different departments elected Ottokar VON CHIARI (1853–1918; M. D. 1877, lecturer 1882, "titular" associate professor 1891, associate professor 1905, "titular" full professor 1907, full professor 1913) as his successor. It was CHIARI who, due to his surgical training under Johann DUMREICHER, (1815–1880) now introduced major surgery in laryngology – first at the laryngological department of the Policlinic and later at the University Clinic of Laryngology. While, for instance, under STOERK for each tracheotomy a surgeon was called in, CHIARI himself performed fissures of the larynx and laryngectomies in his department at the Policlinic.

The first total laryngectomy for cancer, by the way, was performed on December 31, 1873, by Theodor BILLROTH (1829–1894), head of the Second Surgical University Clinic at the Vienna General Hospital. It was a dramatic event which happened there on New Year's Eve, which Karel B. ABSOLON retells: "This is the story of a 36-year-old teacher of theology who had been hoarse for three years. The hoarseness intensified despite cauterization of his vocal cords with silver nitrate and later, intraparenchymatous injections ... In March 1873 a tumor was seen on laryngoscopy, and a diagnosis of malignancy was established. Partial excision of the tumor improved the stenosis and its consequences. Because of its broad basis, it was impossible to remove this tumor endoscopically. The nature of the tumor was clarified by microscopic examination; the clinical course had already suggested its nature. The removal of the cancer which was located under the true vocal cords appeared feasible if the inside of the larynx could be exposed. A laryngotomy was suggested to the patient and on November 21, 1873, he was admitted to Prof. Theodor BILLROTH's clinic. Dr. BILLROTH operated in an attempt to save the left vocal cord, which was not yet involved although the tumor appeared to have spread into the proximal portion

stion"¹¹⁴. Noch mehrmals hat Arthur SCHNITZLER für Aufsehen gesorgt: seine Komödie in fünf Akten ‚Professor Bernhardi' wurde 1913 von der Wiener Zensurbehörde „wegen der zu wahrenden öffentlichen Interessen" verboten und erst 1920 in Wien aufgeführt. Noch im Jahr 1946 erhoben sich warnende Stimmen gegen das politisch brisante Werk, das um eine Affäre kreist, die zwar frei erfunden ist, deren Wirklichkeitsbezüge ohne Zweifel in den Anfeindungen und Kränkungen zu suchen sind, die SCHNITZLERS Vater als Gründungsmitglied und späterer Direktor der Poliklinik erfahren mußte.¹¹⁵
Als um 1890 die ersten Mitteilungen über die Erfolge des KOCHschen Tuberkulins die medizinische Welt im wahrsten Sinne des Wortes in Aufregung versetzten, wurden auch an der Poliklinik sogleich die Versuche damit aufgenommen und in den Jahresberichten darüber sogar mit genauen Krankengeschichten berichtet. Auch Johann SCHNITZLER hat an seiner Abteilung besonders bei Kehlkopftuberkulose Versuche damit angestellt.¹¹⁶
Im Jahr 1892 konnte J. SCHNITZLER noch die Übersiedlung der Poliklinik in das neu erbaute Haus in der Mariannengasse 10 erleben. Die ihm und URBANTSCHITSCH gemeinsam zur Verfügung stehende Abteilung bestand aus einem Wartezimmer, zwei Ordinationsräumen und einem Hörsaal im ersten Stock.
Nach J. SCHNITZLERS Tod fiel die Wahl der Primarii auf Ottokar VON CHIARI (1853–1918), den Schüler und Assistenten SCHRÖTTERS, der 1882 für Laryngologie habilitiert und 1891 zum a. o. Professor ernannt wurde. Dank seiner gründlichen chirurgischen Ausbildung war CHIARI dazu befähigt, auch die größeren chirurgischen Eingriffe an den oberen Luft- und Speisewegen selbständig durchzuführen. Während an der Klinik STOERK noch zu jeder Tracheotomie ein Fachchirurg zugezogen wurde, nahm CHIARI bereits Laryngofissuren und Kehlkopfexstirpationen an der Poliklinik vor.
Die erste Totalexstirpation des Kehlkopfes wurde übrigens am 31. Dezember 1873 von Theodor BILLROTH (1829–1894), dem Vorstand der II. Chirurgischen Universitätsklinik in Wien, bei einem ausgedehnten Larynxkarzinom durchgeführt. Es war ein dramatisches Ereignis, das sich am Silvestertag dieses Jahres im Allgemeinen Krankenhaus abspielte: BILLROTH wollte bei einem 35jährigen Patienten eine Auskratzung des im Kehlkopfbereich gelegenen Tumorgewebes vornehmen. Als der Patient bereits in Narkose war, merkte Billroth, daß selbst diese Operation den baldigen Erstickungstod nicht zu verhindern imstande wäre, und entschloß sich zu der drei Jahre vorher von seinem Schüler Vincenz CZERNY (1842–1916) am Hunde bereits erprobten totalen Kehlkopfresektion. Die Narkose wurde unterbrochen, der Patient um seine Einwilligung befragt und dann die Operation vollendet. Ein anderer Assistent BILLROTHS, Carl GUSSENBAUER (1842–1903), mußte einige Stunden danach eine lebensgefährliche Blutung stillen, und BILLROTH überließ ihm die Publikation¹¹⁷ der erstmals am Menschen durchgeführten Operation.¹¹⁸
Doch zurück zu CHIARI: Seine besondere Bedeutung und sein Verdienst liegen in den erfolgreichen Bemühungen, die Laryngologie, die einst nur ein Nebenfach der inneren Medizin war, selbständig zu machen, ihr die Rhinologie anzugliedern und durch Einbeziehung der Schädel- und Halsoperationen das Fach zu einem vorwiegend chirurgischen auszubauen.
Nach STOERKS Tod wurde CHIARI 1899 als Vorstand an die laryngologische Klinik berufen und benannte diese getreu

of the trachea. The larynx was opened by cutting through the thyroid cartilage. Carl GUSSENBAUER (1842–1903), BILLROTH's assistant reported: '. . . in order to accurately resect the tumor, it was necessary to divide the ring cartilage and was therefore displaced due to the heavy cough of the patient. The trachea was adequately tamponaded with sponges. The cancer was excised with curved scissors. The whole surface was curetted with a sharp spoon and the copious bleeding was stopped by compression.' Formerly, compression and a solution of iron had been the standard application for hemostasis. BILLROTH's laryngotomy procedure accomplished only a partial excision. The day after the operation the patient had been feeling quite well and breathing almost entirely through the larynx. He talked with a low almost toneless voice, but suppuration developed on the second day. He ran a slight temperature which subsided on the fourth day. From then on, scarring of the wound and copious granulations with discharge of necrotic tissue progressed rapidly . . . Laryngoscopic examination on the 16th of December showed a well preserved right vocal cord but a recurrence of the cancer. BILLROTH was somewhat cautious and reluctant to apply a hitherto untried operation, even though the patient was ready to accept 'any type of intervention'. On December 31, the patient was anesthetized through a tracheostomy, the old incision was split, and the fungating cancer visualized. The plan to cauterize this tumor chemically under direct vision was fruitless because of its size. Before BILLROTH had barely half of the larynx opened, he could see the cancer involved the whole mucosa, the internal perichondrium and in the area of the scar even the external perichondrium. He decided to resect the whole larynx as Vincenz CZERNY (1842–1916) had suggested for such otherwise inoperable carcinomas of the inner larynx. Thus, with the more conservative approach eliminated, BILLROTH prepared for the first total laryngectomy for cancer, 'to tear this still young man from the arms of a certain and torturous death.'
The patient was awakened from anesthesia and told of the surgeon's decision! After he gave his consent, the anesthesia was deepened and the first operation of its kind was begun. The incision was made through the soft tissues freeing the larynx on both sides. Scarring from the previous operation increased the difficulty. Two fairly large branches of the superior right thyroid artery bled and were ligated. When the larynx was brought forward with sharp hook retractors, the ring cartilage tore as it was infiltrated and softened by granulation tissue. This limited the retraction considerably and delayed the operative procedure so that the patient awoke. Tracheal aspiration was prevented both by the patient's severe cough and by rapid blotting with sponges.
The patient was re-anesthetized and the larynx again pulled forward with a sharp double-hooked instrument. The ring cartilage was dissected from the anterior surface of the esophagus. GUSSENBAUER noted: 'It was then relatively easy to free the upper end of the cricoid and arytenoid cartilage from the esophagus, isolate the larynx from the back to the front, and finally divide the thyroid ligament. This last part of the operation was accomplished with haste, because of severe bleeding from both superior laryngeal arteries.'¹¹⁷
Two large sponges were placed in the wound and compressed to the side of the neck; when complete hemostasis was accomplished, the sponges were removed. 'The laryngeal mucosa was infiltrated by cancer, which spread into the

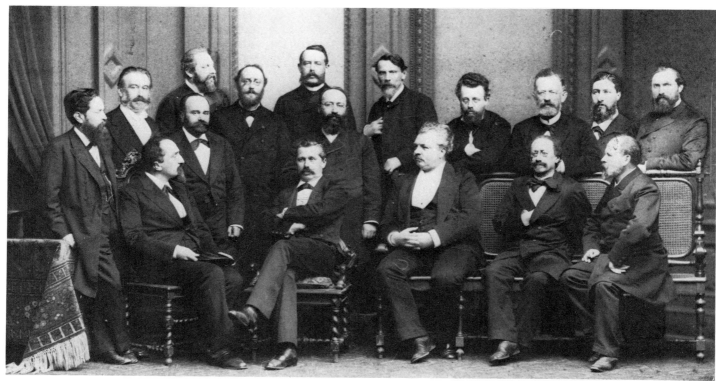

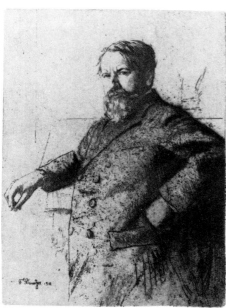

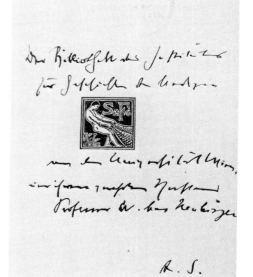

Oben: Das Primarärztekollegium der Poliklinik zwischen 1880 und 1885. Zweiter von links, sitzend: Johann Schnitzler, einer der Mitbegründer der Poliklinik und ihr Direktor von 1884 bis zu seinem Tod im Jahr 1893.
Links unten: Der Schriftsteller-Arzt Arthur Schnitzler. Lithographie von F. Schmutzer, Wien 1912.
Arthur Schnitzler war von 1888–1893 Assistent seines Vaters Johann Schnitzler an der laryngologischen Abteilung der Poliklinik.
Rechts unten: Arthur Schnitzler widmete dieses Exemplar seiner Komödie „Professor Bernhardi" dem damaligen Vorstand des Instituts für Geschichte der Medizin, Max Neuburger. Mit dem Problem des Antisemitismus hat sich Schnitzler in seinem Werk immer wieder auseinandergesetzt, so auch in „Professor Bernhardi", auf dessen Beziehung zu seiner Studienzeit Schnitzler in seiner Autobiographie „Jugend in Wien" hingewiesen hat.

Top: The College of Primarii of the Policlinic between 1880 and 1885. Second from left, seated: Johann Schnitzler, one of the founders of the Policlinic and its director from 1884 until his death in 1893.
Bottom left: The writer-physician Arthur Schnitzler. Lithograph, F. Schmutzer, Vienna, 1912.
Arthur Schnitzler was assistant to his father Johann Schnitzler in the laryngological department of the Policlinic from 1883–1893.
Bottom right: Arthur Schnitzler dedicated this copy of his comedy "Professor Bernhardi" to the Head of the Institute for the History of Medicine at that time, Max Neuburger. Schnitzler repeatedly took issue with anti-Semitism in his oevre, as he does here in "Professor Bernhardi", and to which he refers in his autobiography "Jugend in Wien".

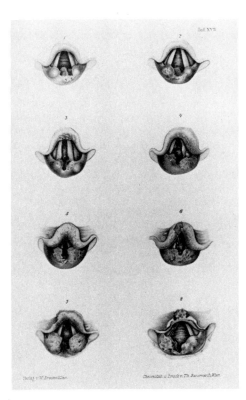

Das Interesse Johann Schnitzlers galt stets auch der Tuberkulosefrage. Als Koch 1890 sein neues Heilverfahren bekanntgab, reiste Schnitzler im selben Jahr nach Berlin, um es dort zu studieren und unternahm im Herbst 1890 an seiner Abteilung der Poliklinik eine Reihe von Versuchen mit dem Kochschen Mittel. Die Berichte und Abbildungen in seinem „Klinischen Atlas der Laryngologie" legen davon Zeugnis ab. Die Figuren 1–8 der Tafel 17 „zeigen ganz ungewöhnlich ausgeprägte Formen von Tuberculose des Kehlkopfes".

Als der Atlas 1895 erschien, war Johann Schnitzler bereits zwei Jahre tot. Das nachgelassene Werk wurde von seinem Sohn Arthur und seinem Assistenten Markus Hajek herausgegeben.

Johann Schnitzler was also interested in tuberculosis. When Koch published his new treatment method in 1890, Schnitzler immediately traveled to Berlin to study the new remedy. In the autumn of the same year, Schnitzler performed a series of experiments in his department with Koch's remedy. The reports and pictures which he published in his "Clinical Atlas of Laryngology" document his interest. Figures 1 to 8 of Table 17 "show unusual manifestations of tuberculosis of the larynx."

This atlas appeared in 1895, two years after Schnitzler's death. It was published by his son Arthur, and his assistant Markus Hajek.

KLINISCHER ATLAS

DER

LARYNGOLOGIE

NEBST ANLEITUNG

ZUR DIAGNOSE UND THERAPIE

DER

KRANKHEITEN DES KEHLKOPFES UND DER LUFTRÖHRE.

HERAUSGEGEBEN

VON

WEIL. Dr. JOH. SCHNITZLER

K. K. REGIERUNGSRATH, PROFESSOR AN DER K. K. UNIVERSITÄT UND DIRECTOR DER ALLGEMEINEN POLIKLINIK IN WIEN

UNTER MITWIRKUNG

VON

Dr. M. HAJEK UND Dr. A. SCHNITZLER

ASSISTENTEN AN DER ALLGEMEINEN POLIKLINIK IN WIEN.

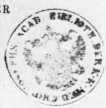

MIT 186 ABBILDUNGEN AUF 28 CHROMOLITH. TAFELN UND 56 HOLZSCHNITTEN IM TEXTE.

WIEN UND LEIPZIG.

WILHELM BRAUMÜLLER

K. u. K. HOF- UND UNIVERSITÄTSBUCHHÄNDLER.

1895.

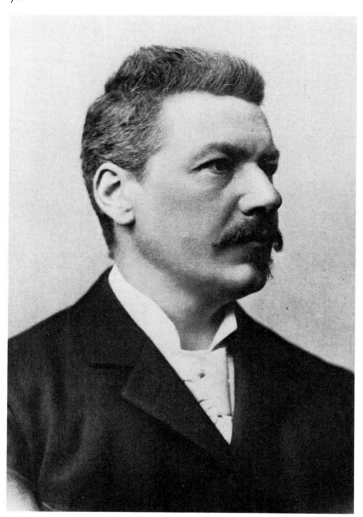

Links: Ottokar von Chiari
Seite 79: Die erste Totalexstirpation des Kehlkopfes wurde am 31. Dezember 1873 von Theodor Billroth (rechts), dem Vorstand der II. Chirurgischen Universitätsklinik in Wien, bei einem ausgedehnten Larynxkarzinom durchgeführt. Billroth überließ die Publikation dieser erstmals am Menschen durchgeführten Operation seinem damaligen Assistenten Carl Gussenbauer. Das linke Bild zeigt den exstirpierten Kehlkopf von oben gesehen: a. Die Begrenzung des Kehlkopfeinganges. b. Das exstirpierte Stück der Epiglottis. c. Die wuchernden Karzinommassen.
(Aus: Gussenbauer, Carl: Über die erste durch Th. Billroth am Menschen ausgeführte Kehlkopf-Exstirpation und die Anwendung eines künstlichen Kehlkopfes. Langenbeck's Archiv für klinische Chirurgie 17 [1874] 343–356.)

Left: Ottokar von Chiari
Page 79: The first total laryngectomy for cancer was performed on December 31, 1873, by Theodor Billroth (right), Head of the Second Surgical University Clinic at the Vienna General Hospital. Billroth's assistant Carl Gussenbauer was given permission to publish the dramatic events of this operation which marked a milestone in surgery.
The picture on the left shows the laryngectomy specimen from above: a. margin of laryngeal entrance; b. resected piece of epiglottis; c. growing mass of cancer.
(From: "Langenbeck's Archives of Clinical Surgery" 17 [1874] 343–356).

seinem Programm in Klinik für Kehlkopf- und Nasenkrankheiten um, wie er auch die Umbenennung der 1895 von STOERK gegründeten Wiener Laryngologischen Gesellschaft in Laryngo-rhinologische Gesellschaft durchsetzte; er sorgte auch dafür, daß die Klinik einen Operationsraum bekam. „Freilich nahm sich dieser anno 1900 noch sehr bescheiden aus. Erst als 1911 die neue, nach den Wünschen CHIARIS und seiner Assistenten Otto KAHLER und Hermann MARSCHIK gebaute Klinik in der Lazarettgasse eröffnet wurde, gab es nicht nur einen, sondern zwei Operationssäle, die mit ihren Spezial-Beleuchtungsreflektoren allen modernen Anforderungen entsprachen. In diesen Räumen hat CHIARI 1912 seine neue Methode der Hypophysenoperation entwickelt. Als er im selben Jahr seine neue Klinik der Öffentlichkeit vorstellte, konnte der sonst so bescheidene Gelehrte sich nicht enthalten zu sagen: ‚Wir glauben, Wien, die Geburtsstadt der klinischen Laryngologie, kann mit Stolz sagen: Die schönste und größte laryngologische Klinik der Welt steht in meinen Mauern.'"119
Als sein Nachfolger übernahm Hans KOSCHIER (1868–1918) im Jahr 1900 die Leitung der laryngologischen Abteilung der Poliklinik. Aus der Schule SCHRÖTTERS hervorgegangen, war KOSCHIER erster Assistent bei STOERK und hatte sich 1898 für Laryngologie habilitiert. Unter KOSCHIER erreichte die von

epiglottis. One third of the latter structure, from its base anterior and to the left, was therefore removed. Part of the upper two tracheal cartilages in proximity of the cancer were resected. The normal mucosa was identified by feel.' One and three quarters of an hour later the trachea was sutured into the skin. Although the patient had lost a 'large amount' of blood and 'suffered much pain', he was 'affected less' than BILLROTH had expected. He was given some wine through a tube and an injection of morphine, and soon fell asleep. A milestone in surgery was complete."118
But let us return to CHIARI: His importance and his achievements lie in his successful efforts to make laryngology – formerly only a branch of internal medicine – an independent specialty, to fuse it with rhinology and to add cranial and cervical surgery, thereby introducing major surgery into laryngology. For this purpose CHIARI needed space. When in 1899 he replaced STOERK as head of the laryngological clinic at the university, he immediately began to press for the construction of a new clinic. The new building, with all modern equipment, was opened in 1911 and CHIARI named it Clinic for Diseases of the Larynx and the Nose, as in 1895 he had changed the name of the Vienna Society for Laryngology, which had been founded by STOERK, to Society for Laryngo-Rhinology. "When the new clinic, which had been built

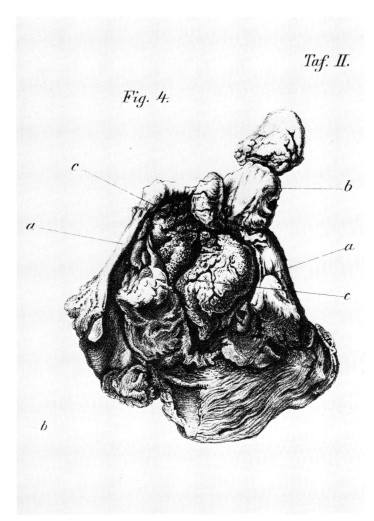

Fig. 4. Taf. II.

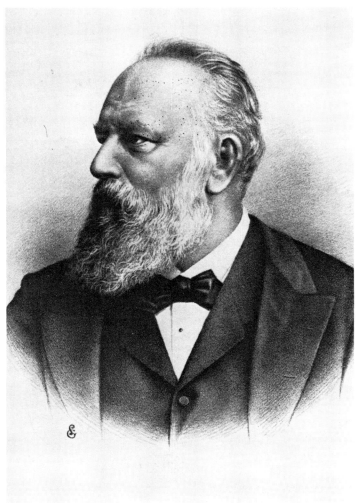

ihm geführte Abteilung einen Höhepunkt ihrer Entwicklung. Mit besonderer Vorliebe arbeitete KOSCHIER an der Verbesserung der Technik der Kehlkopfexstirpation. Seit der Gründung der Anstalt erhielt KOSCHIER als erster eine eigene aus zwei Zimmern bestehende Bettenabteilung. Unter den operativen Eingriffen wurden auch die Septumoperation, die endonasalen Nebenhöhlenoperationen und die 1908 von Amerika aus eingeführte Tonsillektomie immer wieder gelehrt und geübt.

Durch KOSCHIERS große Beliebtheit bei den Wiener Ärzten und seinen Patienten, durch sein erfolgreiches Wirken an der Abteilung stieg die Zahl der pro Jahr behandelten neuen Ambulanzpatienten stetig an, bis im Jahr 1912/13 die Rekordzahl von 8800 Patienten erreicht werden konnte.[120] Die Ambulanzstunden wurden von den Vormittags- auch auf die Nachmittagsstunden ausgedehnt und auch eine Ambulanz an Sonn- und Feiertagen eingeführt. 1911 wurde KOSCHIER zum a. o. Professor ernannt. Nach KOSCHIERS Tod im Jahr 1918 war Josef KAISER unter den schwierigsten Verhältnissen der Nachkriegszeit (Sperre der Bettenstation wegen Kohlenmangels) bemüht, die Abteilung nach dem Vorbild seines Lehrers weiterzuführen.

1920 übernahm dann Hermann MARSCHIK (1878–1969), Oberarzt der Klinik CHIARI und HAJEK, seit 1914 für

according to CHIARI's, and his assistants Otto KAHLER's and Hermann MARSCHIK's wishes, was opened in the Lazarettgasse in 1911, it could boast of two operating theaters, equipped with the most modern devices such as special light-reflectors, etc. In these rooms CHIARI developed his new method of hypophyseal operations in 1912. When in the same year he introduced his new clinic to the public the otherwise very modest CHIARI could not refrain from saying: 'We believe that Vienna, the birth-place of laryngology, can be proud of the most beautiful and largest laryngological clinic in the world which it houses.'"[119]

Hans KOSCHIER (1868–1918) succeeded CHIARI at the Policlinic in 1900. The SCHRÖTTER disciple KOSCHIER had been STOERK's First Assistant and in 1898 had become lecturer in laryngology. The Department of Laryngology at the Policlinic reached the peak of its development under KOSCHIER. His main interest was to improve and perfect the technique of laryngectomies. KOSCHIER was the first one who in the Policlinic's long history was given his own ward with two rooms. KOSCHIER also taught and practiced surgery of septum tumors, endonasal sinus operations and tonsillectomies, which were introduced in 1908 from America.

Due to KOSCHIER's popularity among Vienna's physicians and his patients and due to his successful work at the Policlin-

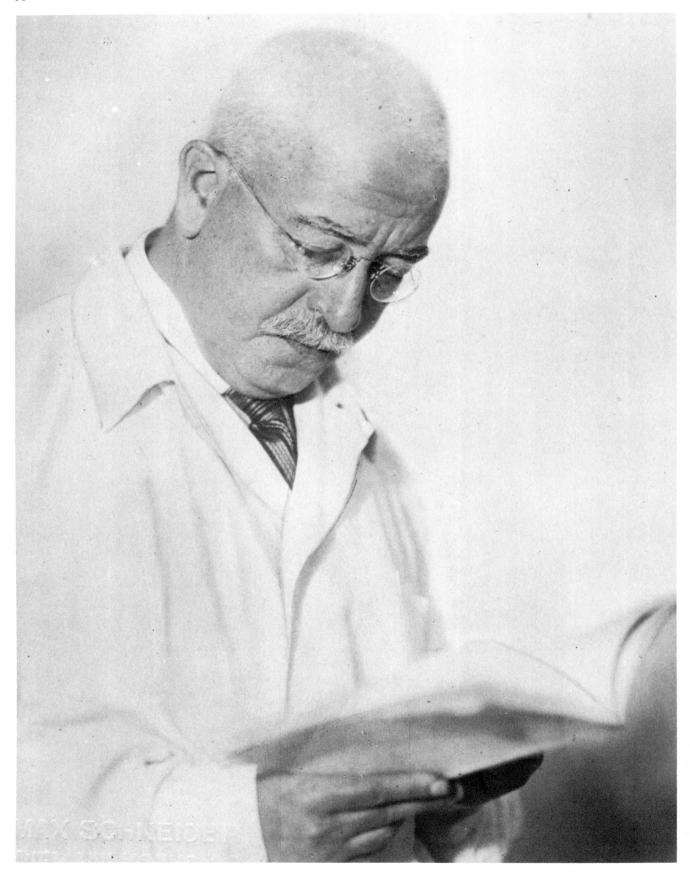

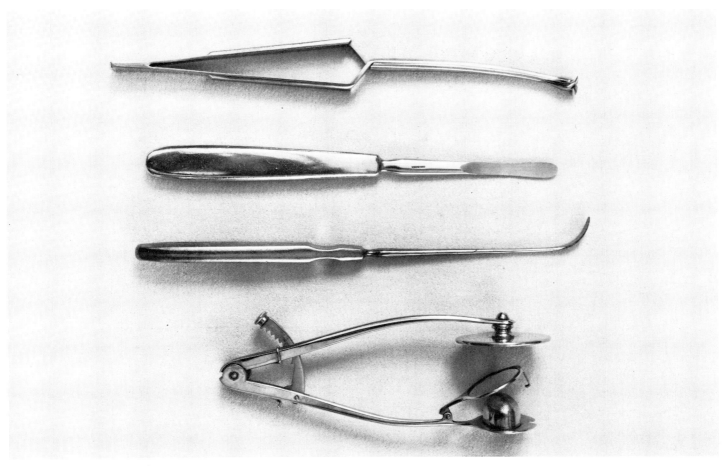

Seite 80: Hermann Marschik

Page 80: Hermann Marschik

Laryngologische Instrumente nach Marschik: Tonsillenfaßpinzette; Tonsillenkompressorium; Tonsillen- und Kieferhöhlenraspatorium.

Laryngological instruments devised by Marschik.

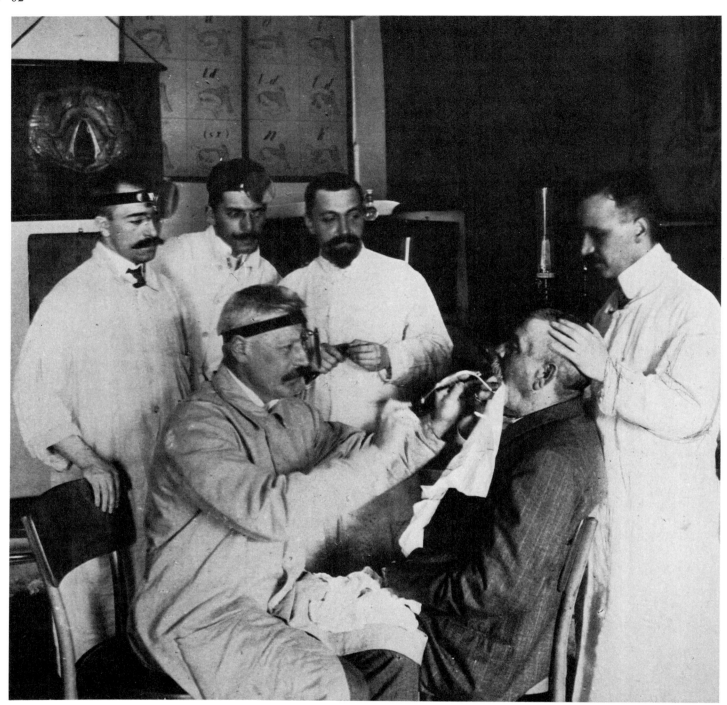

Ottokar von Chiari mit seinen Assistenten Hermann Marschik (hinter ihm) und Otto Kahler (neben ihm) bei einem endolaryngealen Eingriff.

Ottokar von Chiari with his assistants Hermann Marschik (behind him) and Otto Kahler (beside him) performing endolaryngeal work.

Laryngo-Rhinologie habilitiert, die Leitung der Abteilung und erhielt im gleichen Jahr den Titel eines Extraordinarius. Bereits in den ersten Jahren seiner Tätigkeit führte MARSCHIK an seiner Abteilung eine Reihe großer Operationen an Larynx- und Pharynxkarzinomen, Oesophagusdivertikeln, Oberkieferkarzinomen und Hypophysentumoren mit Erfolg durch. Auf Grund seiner im Ersten Weltkrieg gesammelten Erfahrungen wurde die von MARSCHIK angegebene lebensrettende collare Mediastinotomie an zahlreichen Fällen ausgeführt. Dabei war eine Aufnahme der Patienten nach der Operation nur durch das kollegiale Entgegenkommen der anderen Abteilungsvorstände möglich, die noch eigene Bettenstationen hatten. KOSCHIERS frühere laryngologische Bettenstation konnte erst 1922 wieder eröffnet werden. Aber auch von dieser Zeit an mußten sowohl die otologische als auch die laryngologische Abteilung die geringe zur Verfügung stehende Bettenzahl unter sich aufteilen. MARSCHIK bemühte sich von Anfang an, den Ambulanzbetrieb in vollem Umfang weiterzuführen. Seit 1920 hielt MARSCHIK regelmäßig Vorlesungen über Diagnostik und Therapie für Studenten und Ärzte, weiters Kurse über die wichtigsten Operationen und die direkte Endoskopie. Neben zahlreichen wissenschaftlichen Arbeiten über die Pathologie und Therapie maligner Tumoren von Nase, Rachen und Kehlkopf, seinen Arbeiten über die Behandlung von Stenosen der oberen Luftwege, erschien 1927 im Handbuch DENKER-KAHLER seine umfassende Abhandlung über die Verletzungen des Kehlkopfes, der Luftröhre und der Bronchien. 1929 konnte MARSCHIK als Erfüllung eines lange gehegten Wunsches eine nach eigenen Plänen eingerichtete Abteilung im Souterrain der Poliklinik eröffnen. Als Assistenten arbeiteten unter MARSCHIK: E. SUCHANEK, Josef KAISER, W. WEISS-FLORENTIN, F. GENZ, H. SCHWARZ-GLOSSY, R. ZEIDLER, H. STERNBERG, Franz Josef MAYER, E. ERTL, BALLACS, H. SZENES, F. SCHRIMPL und B. GUSIC (später Ordinarius in Zagreb).

Neben seiner medizinischen Tätigkeit war MARSCHIK auch begeisterter Musiker, der Orgel, Viola, Klavier, Pauke und Schlagwerk spielte, und auch Kammermusikwerke und Orchestersuiten – auch für das Wiener Ärzteorchester – komponierte.

Hier soll nun auch ein wenig auf die Verbindung der Wiener Ärzte und insbesondere der Laryngologen mit der Musik eingegangen werden,[121] denn der Dreiklang: Wien – Medizin – Musik ist zweifellos weltweit ein spezifischer Ausdruck österreichischer Kultur.

Leopold SCHRÖTTER VON KRISTELLI war mit Anton BRUCKNER befreundet, den SCHRÖTTER auch behandelte. SCHRÖTTERS Schüler Nikolaus VON JAGIĆ (1875–1956) rühmte SCHRÖTTER als temperamentvollen Geiger. Das bereits genannte Ärzteorchester wurde in Wien im Jahr 1909 von Leopold RÉTHI (1857–1924) gegründet. Der aus Ungarn stammende, 1880 in Wien promovierte Laryngologe war in erster Linie Schüler von Johann SCHNITZLER. SCHNITZLER hatte übrigens seit 1876 eine Professur am Konservatorium für Musik und darstellende Kunst inne und bekleidete diese Stelle bis zu seinem Tod; er hielt dort Vorlesungen über Physiologie und Pathologie der Stimme. RÉTHI, mit einer bekannten Konzertsängerin verheiratet, unterrichtete gleichfalls am Konservatorium, und zwar Stimmphysiologie und Stimmhygiene. Physiologie und Pathologie des Stimmorgans waren zeit seines Lebens RÉTHIS Hauptarbeitsgebiet. In dem von ihm gegründeten Orchester, dessen Präsident er war,

ic the number of out-patients treated every year increased continuously and reached 8,800 in 1912–13.[120] The opening hours of the out-patient department were prolonged. It was now open mornings and afternoons and even on Sundays and public holidays. When KOSCHIER died in 1918, Josef KAISER continued his teacher's work under the most difficult conditions of the post World War One period. For instance, the laryngological ward had to be closed because of lack of coal. In 1920 Hermann MARSCHIK (1878–1969), head-physician under CHIARI and HAJEK and since 1914 lecturer for laryngo-rhinology, became head of the laryngological department of the Policlinic. He was made "titular" associate professor in the same year. Already during the first years of his appointment, MARSCHIK successfully performed major surgical operations of carcinomas of the larynx and pharynx, of the maxilla, esophageal diverticula and tumors of the hypophysis. Due to the experiences he had gathered in World War One he also performed several life-saving cervical mediastinotomies. Since the laryngological ward could not be re-opened until 1922, the patients had to be admitted to other wards for postoperative treatment. From the very beginning, MARSCHIK tried to maintain the entire treatment of ambulatory patients. Since 1920 he also lectured regularly on diagnostics and therapy, held courses in surgical techniques as well as courses on direct endoscopy.

MARSCHIK published a great number of scientific works on the pathology and therapy of malignant tumors of the nose, pharynx and larynx, and on the treatment of stenosis of the larger air-passages. In 1927 his treatise on the lesions of the larynx, trachea and bronchi appeared in the handbook by DENKER-KAHLER.

In 1929 MARSCHIK's greatest wish became reality: he was able to move into the new department of the Policlinic which he himself had planned.

His assistants were: E. SUCHANEK, Josef KAISER, W. WEISS-FLORENTIN, F. GENZ, H. SCHWARZ-GLOSSY, R. ZEIDLER, H. STERNBERG, Franz Josef MAYER, E. ERTL, BALLACS, H. SZENES, F. SCHRIMPL and B. GUSIC who later became full professor in Zagreb (Yugoslavia).

Beside his medical work, MARSCHIK was an enthusiastic and talented musician. He not only played several instruments such as the organ, piano, viola and drums, he also composed chamber and orchestra music – including for the Vienna Orchestra of Physicians.

At this point a few words should be said about the connection between Viennese physicians, particularly the laryngologists, and music, since the combination "Vienna – medicine – music" undoubtedly strikes a harmonic chord reflecting a characteristic expression of Austrian culture.[121]

Leopold SCHRÖTTER VON KRISTELLI was the friend and physician of Anton BRUCKNER. SCHRÖTTER's pupil, Nikolaus VON JAGIĆ (1875–1956) claimed that his teacher was a vivacious violinist. The Orchestra of Physicians was founded in Vienna in 1909 by Leopold RÉTHI (1857–1924). The laryngologist RÉTHI, who came from Hungary and became a doctor of medicine at the University of Vienna in 1880, had primarily studied under Johann SCHNITZLER. Incidentally, since 1876 SCHNITZLER had had a professorship at the Conservatory for Music and the Performing Arts, a position which he kept till his death; he lectured on the physiology and pathology of the larynx. RÉTHI, whose wife was a well-known concert singer, likewise gave instruction at the conservatory in vocal physiol-

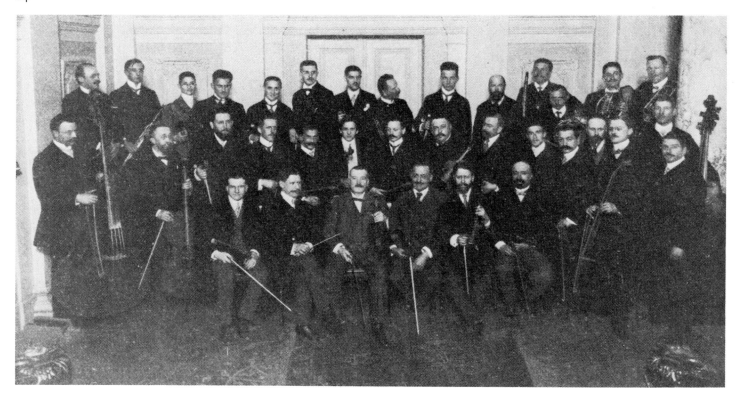

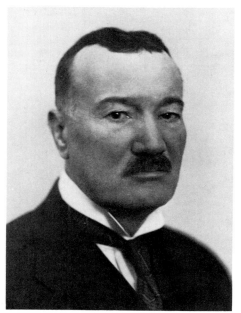
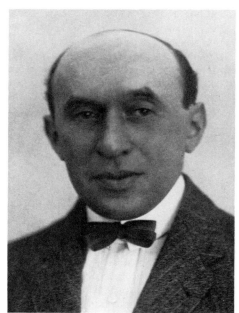

Oben: Die Mitglieder des Wiener Ärzteorchesters im Jahr 1912.
Bildmitte (sitzend): Der Gründer und Präsident des Orchesters Leopold Réthi; links neben ihm: der Dirigent des Orchesters, Nikolaus von Jagić.
Links unten: Leopold Réthi, der 1912 die „Österreichische Gesellschaft für experimentelle Phonetik" gründete.
Rechts unten: Emil Fröschels, Pionier der Logopädie.

Top: The members of the Vienna Orchestra of Physicians in 1912.
Seated in the middle: the founder and president of the orchestra Leopold Réthi; to his left: the conductor Nikolaus von Jagić.
Bottom left: Leopold Réthi, who in 1912 founded the "Austrian Society for Experimental Phonetics".
Bottom right: Emil Fröschels, pioneer of logopedics in Austria.

spielte er Erste Geige. Der Dirigent des Orchesters war seit der Gründung bis zum Jahr 1920 der Internist Nikolaus VON JAGIĆ. Eine Photographie des Orchesters aus dem Jahr 1912 zeigt eine Reihe bedeutender Ärzte, die damals der Vereinigung angehörten. Da spielte z. B. der Medizinstudent Eduard PERNKOPF (1888–1955) Viola, der damalige Dozent Rudolf MARESCH (1868–1936) Zweite Geige, wie auch der Student Fritz PORDES (1890–1936), der später zu Guido HOLZKNECHT (1872–1930) kam. Im April 1923, am Eröffnungstag des 35. Kongresses der Deutschen Gesellschaft für Innere Medizin, spielte dieses Orchester „Wienerisches" im Kursalon des Stadtparks. Am Vormittag eröffnete der Internist Karel Frederik WENCKEBACH (1864–1940) diesen Kongreß mit seinem Vortrag über „Kunst und Medizin". Der darauf folgende Abend aber war ein Ereignis, das wirklich noch einmal die große BILLROTH-BRAHMS- Zeit widerspiegelte: Richard STRAUSS persönlich dirigierte für WENCKEBACH und seine Gäste als Festvorstellung in der Staatsoper seine „Ariadne auf Naxos".

Leopold RÉTHI gründete übrigens 1912 die „Österreichische Gesellschaft für experimentelle Phonetik". Zu dieser Gesellschaft gesellte sich als wertvolles Mitglied der Pionier der eben sich formierenden Logopädie, Emil FRÖSCHELS (1884–1972), und zwar von der otologisch-psychologischen Richtung her. Seine mit dem Lehrer Karl C. ROTHE 1921 begründeten Sprachheilklassen und Kurse leiteten „eine neue Ära in der systematisch und öffentlich geförderten Behandlung der Sprachstörungen ein".[122]

Als Markus HAJEK (1861–1941) seine Monographie über die „Pathologie und Therapie der entzündlichen Erkrankungen der Nebenhöhlen der Nasen" im Jahr 1899 im Druck erscheinen ließ, erfüllte er damit zwei Aufgaben: erstens vollendete er damit für seinen Fachbereich ein Anliegen Carl VON ROKITANSKYS, das freilich noch dem vorigen Jahrhundert angehörte, zweitens aber eröffnete er mit diesem Lehrbuch neue Wege chirurgischer Behandlung, die für die ersten Jahrzehnte unseres Jahrhunderts maßgeblich wurden. Die fünfte Auflage dieses Werkes erschien allerdings erst 1926, und zwar in Amerika. Wie viel stille, ja man möchte sagen, verborgene Arbeit ging diesem Werk voraus!

Schon in seiner ersten Assistentenzeit bei Johann SCHNITZLER an der Poliklinik reifte in HAJEK der Plan, die laryngoskopischen Vorlesungen, bei denen er einen Mangel an topographischer Vorstellungsmöglichkeit bei den Studenten bemerkte, durch Kurse über die Anatomie des Kehlkopfes und der Nase für Kliniker zu ergänzen. SCHNITZLER war damit einverstanden, und es begann für HAJEK eine neunjährige Tätigkeit, in der er durch Lehren selbst lernen konnte. Als er im zehnten Jahre habilitiert wurde, konnte er bereits auf die stattliche Zahl von 1100 Kursteilnehmern zurückblicken; diese setzten sich, der damaligen Zusammensetzung der Hörer an der Wiener Universität entsprechend, „aus allen Ländern der Welt" zusammen, wie HAJEK selbst sagte.[123]

Im Anatomen Emil ZUCKERKANDL (1849–1910) hatte HAJEK das große Vorbild gefunden. Seine „Normale und pathologische Anatomie der Nasenhöhle und ihrer pneumatischen Anhänge" war nicht nur dem Stoff nach seinen eigenen Arbeiten ähnlich, auch die Tendenz ZUCKERKANDLS wurde der Ausgangspunkt für HAJEKS Untersuchungen. Nannte ZUCKERKANDL seine Arbeit eine „Generalstabskarte" für die Operateure, so war des Klinikers HAJEK anatomische Forschung von allem Anfang an auf die klinische Verwertung abgestellt;

ogy and vocal hygiene. Physiology and pathology of the larynx were RÉTHI's special field of interest. In the orchestra which he both initiated and presided over, he played first violin. The conductor from 1909 to 1920 was the internal specialist Nikolaus VON JAGIĆ. A photograph of the orchestra from the year 1912 shows numerous important physicians who belonged to the organization at that time. There was, for instance, the medical student Eduard PERNKOPF (1888–1955) who played viola; Docent Rudolf MARESCH (1868–1936) second violin; and the student Fritz PORDES (1890–1936), who later worked under Guido HOLZKNECHT (1872–1930). On the opening day of the 35th Congress of the German Society for Internal Medicine in April, 1923, this orchestra played "Viennese Specialties" in the Kursalon of the Stadtpark. The internal specialist Karel Frederik WENCKEBACH (1864–1940) gave an opening address that morning with the title "Art and Medicine". But the following evening was an occasion reminiscent of the grand BILLROTH – BRAHMS era: Richard STRAUSS personally conducted a gala performance of his "Ariadne auf Naxos" in the Vienna State Opera for WENCKEBACH and his guests.

Leopold RÉTHI founded the "Austrian Society for Experimental Phonetics" in 1912. A valuable member of this society was the pioneer of the fledgling field of logopedics Emil FRÖSCHELS (1884–1972), who approached the new discipline from a background of otological-psychology. The classes and courses in speech pathology and therapy which he originated with the teacher Karl C. ROTHE in 1921 paved the way for "a new era in the systematic and publicly supported treatment of speech defects."[122]

When Markus HAJEK (1861–1941; M. D. 1879, lecturer 1879, "titular" associate professor 1912, "titular" full professor 1919) published his monograph on the "Pathology and Therapy of Inflammatory Diseases of the Sinus and Nasal Passages" in 1899, he fulfilled two tasks: First, he completed the unfinished business of Carl VON ROKITANSKY with regard to his discipline, albeit a concern of the previous century; and second, with this text he opened the way for a new surgical treatment which was to become decisive for the first decades of our century. The fifth edition of this work did not appear until 1926, and that was in America. But how much silent – one must almost say hidden – work went into this book! When he was an assistant under Johann SCHNITZLER at the Policlinic HAJEK devised a plan to supplement the lectures on laryngoscopy – in which HAJEK noticed a lack on the part of the students of the capacity to imagine topographical features – with courses on the anatomy of the larynx and nose. SCHNITZLER approved of the proposal, so HAJEK began a nine-year period during which he was to learn himself through teaching. When he became lecturer in his tenth year, he could look back at the impressive number of 1,100 course participants; they came "from all the countries in the world", as HAJEK said himself,[123] which was consistent with other enrollments at the University of Vienna at the time.

The anatomist Emil ZUCKERKANDL (1849–1910) had been HAJEK's ideal. His "Normal and Pathological Anatomy of the Nasal Cavity and Its Pneumatic Appendices" (Vienna, 1882) was not only similar to his publications in substance; ZUCKERKANDL's tendency was also the starting point for HAJEK's research. If ZUCKERKANDL called his work a "map for the operating joint chiefs of staff", the clinician HAJEK's anatomical research was directed towards the clinical aspects

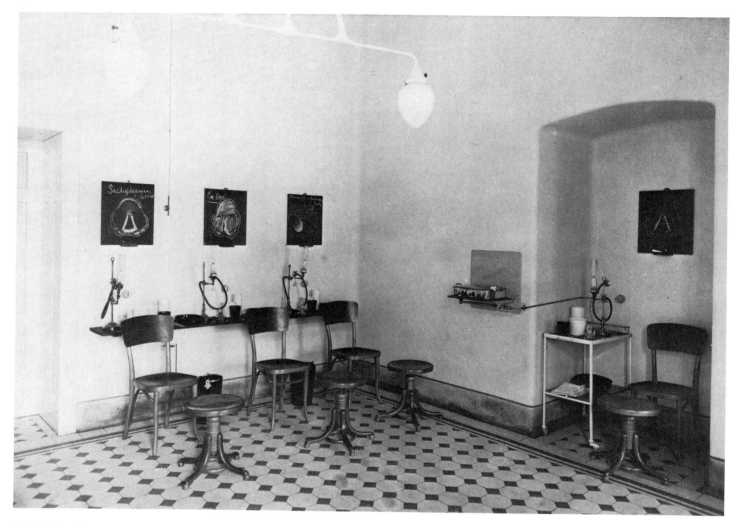

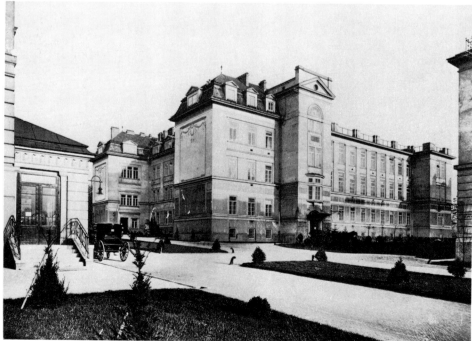

Oben: Behandlungsraum der Klinik.
Unten: Die neue, 1911 eröffnete Klinik für Kehlkopf- und Nasenkrankheiten in Wien IX., Lazarettgasse 14. Als Ottokar von Chiari 1912 die nach seinen Wünschen geplante und gebaute Klinik der Öffentlichkeit vorstellte, sagte er: „Wir glauben, Wien, die Geburtsstadt der klinischen Laryngologie, kann mit Stolz sagen: Die schönste und größte laryngologische Klinik der Welt steht in meinen Mauern."

Top: Surgery of the new clinic.
Bottom: The new Clinic for Diseases of the Larynx and the Nose in Vienna's ninth district, Lazarettgasse 14. When in 1912 Ottokar von Chiari introduced his new clinic to the public he said: "We believe that Vienna, the birth-place of laryngology, can be proud of the most beautiful and largest laryngological clinic in the world which it houses."

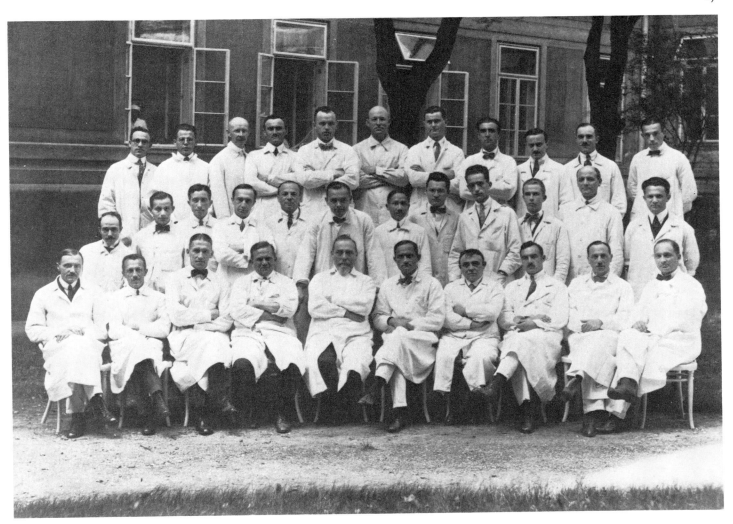

Oben: Markus Hajek (Bildmitte, sitzend) mit seinen Assistenten vor seiner Klinik.
Unten: Markus Hajek, sitzend, mit Stirnreflektor, bei der Untersuchung einer Patientin im Kreise seiner Mitarbeiter: E. G. Mayer, Leidler, Waldapfel, Haslinger, Hofer, Wiethe, Großmann, Stern, Wessely, Heindl.
Nach einer Zeichnung von M. Schneider, Wien 1931.

Top: Seated in the middle is Markus Hajek, surrounded by the assistants at his clinic.
Bottom: Markus Hajek (seated with head-reflector) examining a patient, surrounded by his staff: E. G. Mayer, Leidler, Waldapfel, Haslinger, Hofer, Wiethe, Großmann, Stern, Wessely, Heindl.
After a drawing by M. Schneider, Vienna, 1931.

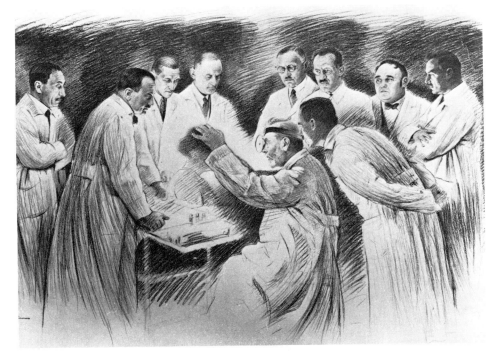

er erfand zahlreiche Spezialinstrumente bzw. entwickelte andere weiter, so daß er mit Recht als „Vater der endonasalen Chirurgie"[124] bezeichnet werden darf.

Ein Grund, warum HAJEKS Lehrbuch durch die ersten drei Jahrzehnte unseres Jahrhunderts seine volle Aktualität behielt, liegt gewiß auch in der Darstellungsweise. Überall merkt man die Frische, entweder überhaupt eigener Forschung, oder unmittelbarer eigener Beobachtung. „Was ich nicht selbst gesehen oder erfahren, betrachte ich nicht als mein geistiges Eigentum." Dieses Motto, das zu HAJEKS 70. Geburtstag einer seiner Schüler, der damalige Grazer Ordinarius Gustav HOFER, 1931 in den Vordergrund stellte,[125] findet man bereits auf jeder Seite seiner Monographie bestätigt. Auch die an HAJEK in späterer Zeit von seinen Hörern so gerühmte instruktive Form des Lehrens, die das Verstehen leicht machte, findet man in dem Werk, das er mit 38 Jahren bereits fertiggestellt hatte, angedeutet. Die Form: knappe, anschaulich geschilderte Krankengeschichten, gut begründete Fehlschlüsse, Richtigstellung des Fehlschlusses und Aufklärung des Problems hatte wohl zu allen Zeiten großen didaktischen Wert. HAJEK besaß bald einen internationalen Ruf, und als sich nach CHIARIS Tod (1918) Anton VON EISELSBERG (1860–1939), ehemals BILLROTHS Schüler, der seines Lehrers Erbe im 20. Jahrhundert würdig und erfolgreich weiter entwickelte, bei der Frage nach der Nachfolge an KILLIAN in Freiburg wandte, erhielt er von diesem die Antwort: „Warum fragen Sie bei mir an, wo Sie doch in Wien einen HAJEK haben."[126] So trat Markus HAJEK 1919 die Nachfolge Ottokar CHIARIS an. HAJEK konnte gerade in dieser Berufung die volle Anerkennung seiner Fachgenossen für seine Bestrebungen erkennen. Zahlreiche Spezialinstrumente entwickelte HAJEK für die Nebenhöhlenchirurgie, und er war der erste, der die Keilbeinhöhle von der Nase her eröffnete. Noch in seiner Antrittsrede, so meint Erna LESKY, spüre man den ganzen Schwung, der den Pionier von damals erfüllte: „Das war eine Zeit der Begeisterung, welche nach wenigen Jahren herrliche Fortschritte zeitigte. Im raschen Fluge erkannten wir nicht nur die Krankheiten der Nasenhöhlenwände, sondern drangen auch in die Nebenhöhlen; zuerst die Kieferhöhle, dann endonasal in die Stirnhöhle, wenige Jahre später legten wir das Siebbeinlabyrinth und die Keilbeinhöhle frei."[127]

Für sein weiteres Schaffen stand HAJEK nun die schon genannte, 1911 unter Mitwirkung CHIARIS gebaute Neue Klinik in Wien IX, Lazarettgasse 14, zur Verfügung. Auf diese Klinik kam am 10. April 1924, auf der vorletzten Station seines Lebensweges, ein Patient, dessen Lebenswerk heute in der Weltliteratur einen festen Platz einnimmt: der am 3. Juli 1883 in Prag geborene Franz KAFKA.[128] Doch auch hier, auf der damals „schönsten und größten laryngologischen Klinik der Welt", die „über die modernsten Einrichtungen"[129] verfügte, konnte man KAFKA nicht mehr helfen: am 19. April 1924 wurde er auf eigenen Wunsch in häusliche Pflege entlassen, „was als letzte Eintragung seiner Krankengeschichte das Ende der anfangs vielversprechenden Behandlung in der schönsten laryngologischen Klinik der Welt bedeutet."[130] – Doch KAFKA fuhr nicht nach Hause: am 19. April 1924 trat er seine letzte Reise in das Privatsanatorium Dr. HOFFMANN in Kierling bei Klosterneuburg an; dort starb er am 3. Juni 1924 an Kehlkopftuberkulose.

Seit den Tagen von TÜRCK und CZERMAK war es das vornehmste Anliegen der Wiener Laryngologie, normale Anato-

from the very beginning. He invented numerous special instruments or developed the existing ones further, so that he may be rightly called "the father of endonasal surgery."[124] One reason why HAJEK's textbook remained current even throughout the first decades of the 20th century lies in the way the subject-matter is presented. The liveliness of the presentation which stems from HAJEK's own research or own observation is felt on each page. "What I have not seen myself or experienced myself, I do not regard as my intellectual property." This motto, which became the center of Gustav HOFER's paper[125] dedicated to HAJEK on the occasion of the latter's 70th birthday in 1931, is proven on each page of HAJEK's monograph. This work also gives ample proof of the author's instructive way of teaching for which he was later praised by his students: brief, instructive case histories, well-substantiated errors of judgement, corrections and explanations of the errors. Such a method has and will certainly always be of great didactic value.

HAJEK soon had an international reputation. When after CHIARI's death (1918) Anton VON EISELSBERG (1860–1939), the former disciple of Theodor BILLROTH, asked Gustav KILLIAN in Freiburg to name a successor to CHIARI, KILLIAN answered: "Why are you asking me, when you have a HAJEK in Vienna."[126] Thus HAJEK succeeded Ottokar CHIARI in 1919. In this appointment HAJEK could see his colleagues' full approval of his work. HAJEK invented numerous special instruments or developed the existing ones further, and he was the first one who opened the sphenoid sinus from the nose. His inaugural lecture reflects this pioneer's élan according to Erna LESKY: "This was a period of enthusiasm, which brought about a rapid progress in our specialty. We not only diagnosed the diseases of the walls of the nasal cavity, we also entered the sinuses. First the sinus maxillaris, then endonasally the sinus frontalis, only a few years later we exposed the ethmoidal labyrinth and the sphenoid sinus."[127]

For his further work HAJEK now had at his disposal the already mentioned Clinic for Diseases of the Larynx and the Nose in Vienna's ninth district, Lazarettgasse 14. In this clinic, on April 10, 1924, a patient was admitted on the next to the last stop of his life: Franz KAFKA, born in Prague on July 3, 1883, whose literary œuvre occupies an eminent position in world-literature.[128] But even there, in the world's "most beautiful and largest laryngological clinic" with the "most modern equipment"[129] there was no help for KAFKA. On April 19, 1924, he left the clinic at his own request to go home, which "as the last entry into his case history also marks the end of an originally promising treatment."[130] – KAFKA did not go home, however: on April 19, 1924 he began his last journey to Dr. HOFFMANN's private sanatorium in Klosterneuburg/Kierling close to Vienna where he died on June 3, 1924, of tuberculosis of the larynx.

Since the days of TÜRCK and CZERMAK it had been the noblest concern of Viennese laryngologists to fuse and teach normal anatomy, pathological anatomy and surgery with endoscopic methods.[131] HAJEK knew how to combine both brilliantly. Equally important is the fact that he also tried not to lose the connection with general medicine. When in 1929 he was given the honor of holding the Semon-lecture in London he chose as topic for his lecture: "Laryngo-Rhinology and General Medicine". HAJEK like so many others was not spared the bitterness of emigration. At the age of 77 he left his beloved Vienna for London where he died in 1941.

Die erste Seite der Krankengeschichte des Prager Schriftstellers Franz Kafka, der im Jahr 1924, kurz vor seinem Tod, zur Behandlung seiner Kehlkopftuberkulose an die Klinik Hajek kam.
Photographie aus dem Privatbesitz von Frau R. Hackermüller, Wien.

*The first page of the case history of the writer Franz Kafka, born in Prague. He came to the Hajek clinic in 1924, shortly before his death, for the treatment of tuberculosis of the larynx.
Photograph in the private collection of Frau R. Hackermüller, Vienna.*

K.

1924.

Laryngologische Klinik.

Prot.-Nr. 135   Z.-Nr. 3

Tag der Aufnahme: 10 April 24

Name: Dr Kafka Franz

Alter, Stand, Beschäftigung: 41 J. Beamter in P. led. mos.

Geburtsort und derzeitiger Wohnort: Prag Altstadter ring 6.

Diagnose: tbc. laryngis

Anatom. od. mikroskop. Befund exstirp. Teile:

Ausgang der Behandlung und Tag des Abganges: Entl. am 19. IV. 1924

Datum	
	Familienanamnese: Sämmtliche Familienangehörigen gesund, keine Tbc. Kinderkrankheiten: Keuchhusten.
	Pat. war immer schwächlich u. sehr zart gebaut, fühlte sich aber ziemlich gesund.
	Vor 6 Jahren Blutsturz, es wurde eine Lungentbc diagnostiziert. Das Lungenleiden wechselt im Laufe der Jahre an Intensität. Pat. hat Zeiten, in denen er sehr gut aussieht u. sich relativ wohl fühlt. In den letzten 7 Monaten hat der Pat. ca 6 kg abgenommen u. fühlt sich jetzt schlechter als während der vergangenen Jahre.
	Vor 2 Wochen wurde Pat. heiser. Seit 5 Tagen bestehen brennende Schmerzen beim Schlucken besonders rechts, oft auch unabhängig davon, die ihn manchmal aus dem Schlafe wecken.

N. Nr. 949 — SALZER IN WIEN

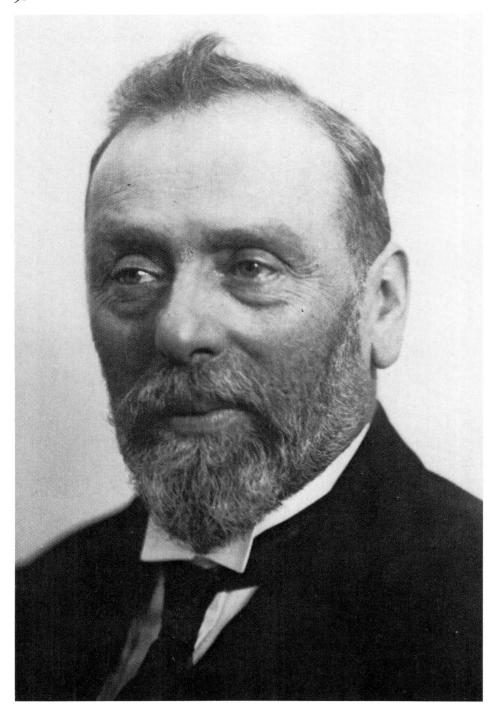
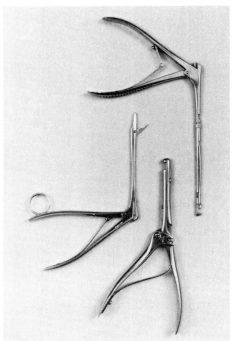
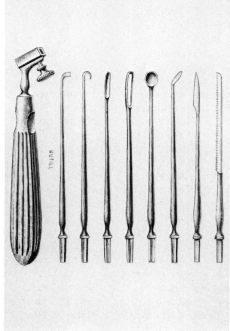

Markus Hajek,
der „Vater der endonasalen Chirurgie".
Photographie von M. Schneider, Wien 1922.

*Markus Hajek,
the "father of endonasal surgery."
Photograph by M. Schneider, Vienna, 1922.*

Rechts oben: Instrumente zur endonasalen Operation nach Hajek.

Top right: Instruments for endonasal operations devised by Markus Hajek.

Rechts unten: Spezialinstrumente nach Hajek zur Siebbeinoperation.

Bottom right: Instruments for ethmoidal operations devised by Markus Hajek.

mie, pathologische Anatomie und Chirurgie mit den endoskopischen Methoden[131] zu vereinen und zu lehren. HAJEK hat beides in meisterhafter Weise verstanden, dazu kam noch, daß er auch darauf bedacht war, den Zusammenhang mit der Allgemeinmedizin nicht zu verlieren. Als ihm 1929 die Ehre zuteil wurde, in London die Semon-Lecture zu halten, wählte er dafür das Thema: „Laryngo-Rhinology and General Medicine". Es blieb HAJEK nicht erspart, aus seinem geliebten Wien vertrieben zu werden: siebenundsiebzigjährig trat er die Flucht an; 1941 starb er in der Londoner Emigration.
Von Franz HASLINGER (Wien) stammt das bekannte Endoskopiebesteck, das sich auch jetzt noch bei der Ösophagoskopie bewährt. Durch zahlreiche Operationen bei intrasellaren Hypophysentumoren mit seiner transseptalen, transsphenoidalen Operationsmethode hat Oskar HIRSCH dem rhinochirurgischen Weg weltweite Anerkennung erworben.
Die Entwicklung nach HAJEK skizziert Otto NOVOTNY (geb. 1911), der von 1954 bis zu seiner Emeritierung im Jahr 1982 die II. Universitäts-Klinik für Hals-, Nasen- und Ohrenkrankheiten leitete: „An der II. HNO-Klinik folgte auf HAJEK Emil WESSELY[132] (1887–1954), nach ihm Camillo WIETHE bis zu dessen Tod (1949), worauf WESSELY noch einmal mit der Leitung betraut wurde. Am 22. September 1954 übernahm ich als ao. Professor die Klinik zunächst supplierend, im Februar 1961 wurde ich zum o. Professor und Leiter der Klinik ernannt. Seit 1970 gibt es wieder zwei HNO-Kliniken. . . . Ich glaube nicht, daß meine Klinik besondere spezielle Methoden entwickelt hat, aber die Leistung seit WESSELY liegt vor allem in der Verfeinerung der Mikrochirurgie. . . . Die Mikrochirurgie hat die operative Ohrenheilkunde wesentlich verändert. . . . Dadurch ist alles viel exakter geworden. . . . Im übrigen liegen unsere Leistungen auf dem Gebiet der Lärmforschung, der Schwerhörigenfürsorge und der Pollenallergie."[133]
Nach NOVOTNY übernahm 1983 Klaus EHRENBERGER (geb. 1938) die Leitung der Klinik.
Die chirurgischen Methoden der Karzinomtherapie hat Johannes ZANGE als Chef der GRAZER Klinik ausgebaut und damals bereits die systematische Ausräumung der Halslymphknoten bei Karzinommetastasen ausgeführt, die nach dem Zweiten Weltkrieg erst von Amerika aus als Neckdissection auch in Europa meist routinemäßig angewendet wird. Mit der Bakteriologie und Serologie der Ozaena beschäftigte sich Gustav HOFER schon als Assistent bei CHIARI frühzeitig. Nach experimenteller Erzeugung der Ozaena beim Tier gelangen ihm erstmalig durch Vakzination auch Heilungen bei Patienten. Neben seinen Arbeiten über die sensible Kehlkopfinnervation konnte HOFER 1937 als Vorstand der Grazer Klinik gemeinsam mit Josef JESCHEK durch experimentelle Nervendurchschneidungen einen wesentlichen Beitrag zur Klärung der motorischen Kehlkopfinnervation liefern. Walter MESSERKLINGER (geb. 1920) hat wegweisende Untersuchungen über die Funktion und den Aufbau der Nasenschleimhäute durchgeführt und die von ihm entwickelten mikroskopischen Untersuchungstechniken der Nase und der Nebenhöhlen vervollkommnet. („Endoscopy of the nose", erschienen 1978 bei Urban-Schwarzenberg, Baltimore–München.)
Ludwig HÖRBST hat nach dem Zweiten Weltkrieg an der INNSBRUCKER Klinik die Röntgenkontaktbestrahlung des Kehlkopfkarzinoms durch ein Schildknorpelfenster ausgearbeitet.

Franz HASLINGER of Vienna developed the well-known endoscopic set of instruments which are still used today for esophagoscopy.
Oskar HIRSCH won himself world-wide recognition due to his numerous operations of intrasellar hypophyseal tumors, for which he developed a special technique.
The development after HAJEK in Vienna is summed up by Otto NOVOTNY (born in 1911), who from 1954 until his retirement in 1982 headed the Second University Clinic for Diseases of the Throat, Nose and Ear: "At the Second ENT-Clinic HAJEK was succeeded by Emil WESSELY (1887–1954),[132] who was followed by Camillo WIETHE. When WIETHE died in 1949 WESSELY was called in again. On September 22, 1954, I was appointed substitute head of the clinic and was given the title associate professor. In February 1961 I became full professor and head of the clinic. Since 1970 there have been again two ENT-clinics . . . I do not believe that my clinic has developed special methods. Its achievements since WESSELY lie in the refinement of micro-surgery, and in the field of noise research, helping the deaf, and pollinoses."[133]
In 1983 Klaus EHRENBERGER (born in 1938) became head of the clinic.
The surgical methods of carcinoma therapy were explored and enlarged by Johannes ZANGE, head of the University Clinic in GRAZ. He propagated the systematic removal of cervical lymph-nodes due to carcinomatosis, which was introduced routinely in Europe from the United States only after World War Two. This method became known as "Neckdissection".
As CHIARI's assistant Gustav HOFER carried out research on the bacteriology and serology of ozaena. After experimentally producing ozaena in animals he was the first one who successfully vaccinated against and cured patients of this disease. Apart from his work on sensory innervation of the larynx, in 1937 HOFER together with Josef JESCHEK was able to make a substantial contribution to the clarification of motor larynx innervation. Walter MESSERKLINGER (born in 1920) carried out pioneering research on the function and constitution of the mucosa of the nose and perfected microscopic techniques for examining the nose and the sinuses, which he himself had developed. His monograph "Endoscopy of the Nose" appeared in 1978.
In INNSBRUCK after World War Two Ludwig HÖRBST pioneered x-ray treatment of carcinomas of the larynx and devised his special technique.

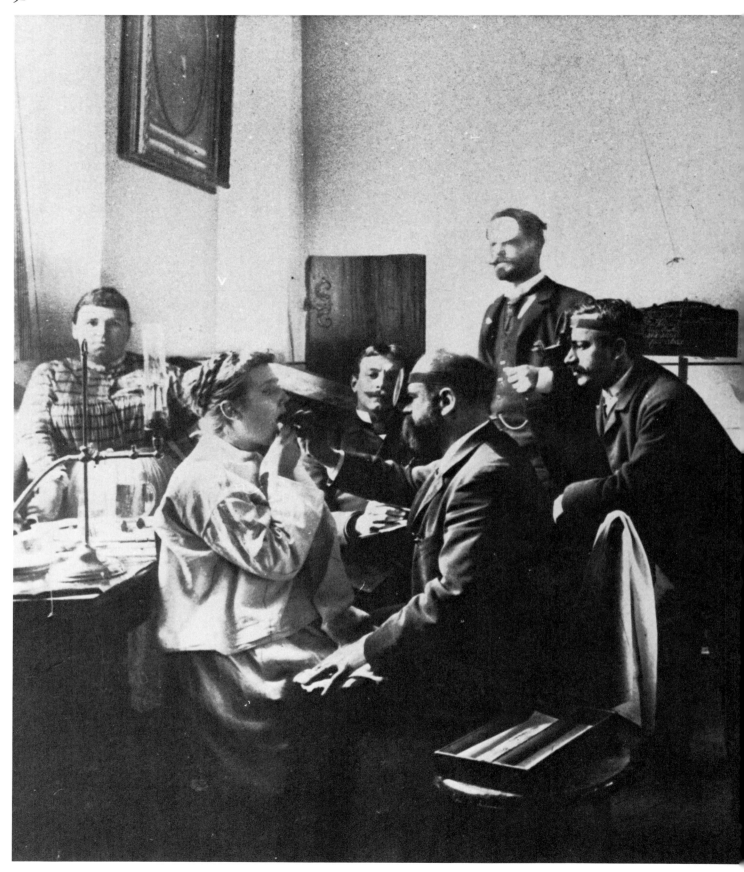

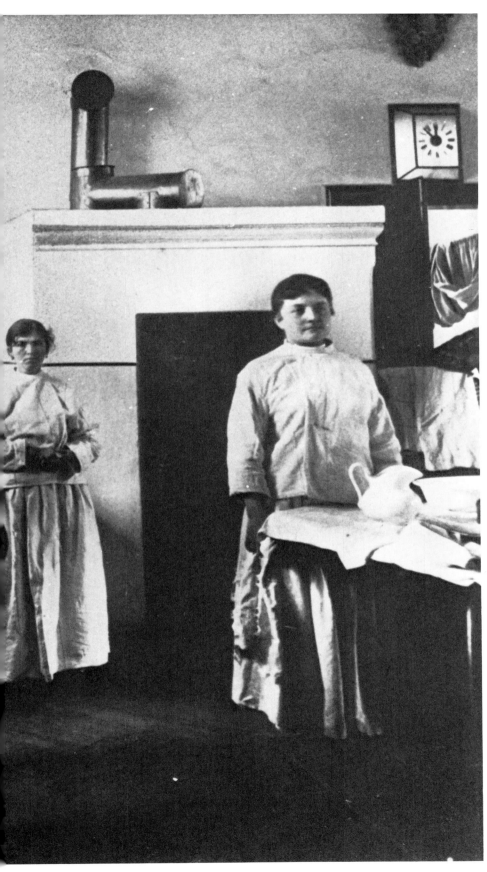

Wie an der Ohrenklinik oder der Ohrenabteilung der Poliklinik wurden auch an der laryngologischen Klinik und der laryngologischen Abteilung der Poliklinik Kurse für ausländische Ärzte abgehalten. Diese Kurse „dauerten meistens sechs Wochen und kosteten 20 Gulden" (Lesky). Die Photographie stammt von Dr. med. Max Köhler und wurde um 1900 aufgenommen. Damals untersuchten die Ärzte noch in Straßenkleidung und bei Gasbeleuchtung.

As at the Clinic of Otology or at the otological department of the Policlinic, courses were also held for foreign physicians at the Clinic of Laryngology and the laryngological department of the Policlinic. These courses "usually lasted six weeks and cost 20 florin" (Lesky). The photograph belonged to Dr. Max Köhler and was taken around 1900. At that time physicians conducted their examinations in street-clothes and by gaslight.

ANMERKUNGEN
REFERENCES

[1] BRESGEN, Maximilian: Die Bedeutung der Arbeitstheilung besonders in der praktischen Medizin. . . . Wiener Medizinische Presse 24 (1883) 247–254, 285–289, 311–315, 343–346, 381–384; 287–288.

[2] BRESGEN, M.: Zur Vereinigung der Otologie mit der Rhino-Laryngologie zu einem einzigen Specialfache. Deutsche Medicinische Wochenschrift 9 (1883) 721.

[3] EULNER, Hans-Heinz: Die Entwicklung der medizinischen Spezialfächer an den Universitäten des deutschen Sprachgebietes. (= Studien zur Medizingeschichte des neunzehnten Jahrhunderts, Bd. IV) Stuttgart 1970, S. 347–386.

[4] MATZKER, Joseph: Zur Entstehungsgeschichte der Oto-Rhino-Laryngologie. Hippokrates 33 (1962) 423–430; 430.

[5] GOETHE, J. W.: Über Naturwissenschaft. Sprüche in Prosa. Goethes sämtliche Werke. Neu durchges. u. erg. Ausg. in 36 Bdn. Mit Einl. v. Karl GOEDEKE. Stuttgart, o. J., Bd. 4, S. 202.

[6] Mit der Diskussion um die Zusammengehörigkeit der HNO-Heilkunde als Spezialfach beschäftigt sich auch u. a. LEICHER, H.: Wandlungen in der Hals-Nasen-Ohrenheilkunde im Lebenslauf eines 82jährigen Klinikers. HNO-Informationen 9 (1984) 27–57.

[7] Vgl. etwa SCHADEWALDT, Hans: Bemerkungen eines Medizinhistorikers zur Entwicklung der Hals-, Nasen-, Ohren-Heilkunde. HNO-Informationen 4 (1979) 13–29, oder BERENDES, J.: Hals-Nasen-Ohrenheilkunde in Deutschland gestern, heute, morgen. HNO-Informationen 8 (1983) 21–25; 21.

[8] SCHADEWALDT, Zit. Anm. 7, S. 26.

[9] O'CONNELL, C. D.: Birth and growth of a speciality. Irish Journal of medical Sciences, Ser. 6, Nr. 401 (1959) 217–227.

[10] Rede des Prof. A. POLITZER bei seinem Rücktritte vom Lehramte gehalten an der Ohrenklinik anläßlich der Abschiedsfeier 1. Oktober 1907. Wiener klinische Wochenschrift 20 (1907) 1327–1329; 1327.

[11] LESKY, Erna: Meilensteine der Wiener Medizin. Große Ärzte Österreichs in drei Jahrhunderten. Wien–München–Bern 1981, S. 189.

[12] PUSCHMANN, Theodor: Die Medicin in Wien während der letzten 100 Jahre. Wien 1884, S. 306.

[13] ARLT, Ferdinand: Meine Erlebnisse. Wiesbaden 1887, S. 63 f.

[14] Zit. Anm. 10, S. 1327.

[15] Zit. Anm. 13, S. 42 f.

[16] LESKY, Erna: Die Wiener medizinische Schule im 19. Jahrhundert. Graz–Köln, 2. Aufl., 1978, S. 220.

[17] Nekrolog Dr. Ignaz GRUBER. Archiv für Ohrenheilkunde 7 (1873) 59–63; 60 f.

[18] Vgl. POLITZER, Adam: Rückblick auf den Fortschritt der Otologie im letzten Jahrhundert. Wiener Medizinische Wochenschrift 39 (1913) 2521–2528; 2521.

[19] STEFAN, J. im Almanach der kaiserlichen Akademie der Wissenschaften 29 (1879) 147–172; 153 f.

---

[1] BRESGEN, Maximilian: Die Bedeutung der Arbeitstheilung besonders in der praktischen Medizin . . . Wiener Medizinische Presse 24 (1883) 247–254, 285–289, 311–315, 343–346, 381–384; 287–288.

[2] BRESGEN, M.: Zur Vereinigung der Otologie mit der Rhino-Laryngologie zu einem einzigen Specialfache. Deutsche Medicinische Wochenschrift 9 (1883) 721.

[3] EULNER, Hans-Heinz: Die Entwicklung der medizinischen Spezialfächer an den Universitäten des deutschen Sprachgebietes. (= Studien zur Medizingeschichte des neunzehnten Jahrhunderts, vol. IV) Stuttgart, 1970, pp. 347–386.

[4] MATZKER, Joseph: Zur Entstehungsgeschichte der Oto-Rhino-Laryngologie. Hippokrates 33 (1962) 423–430; 430.

[5] GOETHE, J. W.: Über Naturwissenschaft. Sprüche in Prosa. Goethes sämtliche Werke. Neu durchges. u. erg. Ausg. in 36 Bdn. Mit Einl. v. Karl GOEDEKE. Stuttgart, n. d., vol. 4, p. 202.

[6] This question is also discussed for instance by LEICHER, H.: Wandlungen in der Hals-Nasen-Ohrenheilkunde im Lebenslauf eines 82jährigen Klinikers. HNO-Informationen 9 (1984) 27–57.

[7] Cf. for instance SCHADEWALDT, Hans: Bemerkungen eines Medizinhistorikers zur Entwicklung der Hals-, Nasen-, Ohren-Heilkunde. HNO-Informationen 4 (1979) 13–29, or BERENDES, J.: Hals-Nasen-Ohrenheilkunde in Deutschland gestern, heute, morgen. HNO-Informationen 8 (1983) 21–25; 21.

[8] SCHADEWALDT, cited in reference 7, p. 26.

[9] O'CONNELL, C. D.: Birth and growth of a speciality. Irish Journal of medical Sciences, Ser. 6, Nr. 401 (1959) 217–227.

[10] Rede des Prof. A. POLITZER bei seinem Rücktritte vom Lehramte gehalten an der Ohrenklinik anläßlich der Abschiedsfeier am 1. Oktober 1907. Wiener klinische Wochenschrift 20 (1907) 1327–1329; 1327.

[11] LESKY, Erna: Meilensteine der Wiener Medizin. Große Ärzte Österreichs in drei Jahrhunderten. Vienna–Munich–Berne, 1981, p. 189.

[12] PUSCHMANN, Theodor: Die Medicin in Wien während der letzten 100 Jahre. Vienna, 1884, p. 306.

[13] ARLT, Ferdinand: Meine Erlebnisse. Wiesbaden, 1887, p. 63 f.

[14] Cited in reference 10, p. 1327.

[15] Cited in reference 13, p. 42 f.

[16] LESKY, Erna: The Vienna Medical School of the 19th Century. The Johns Hopkins University Press. Baltimore and London, 1976, p. 192.

[17] Nekrolog Dr. Ignaz GRUBER. Archiv für Ohrenheilkunde 7 (1873) 59–63; 60 f.

[18] Cf. POLITZER, Adam: Rückblick auf den Fortschritt der Otologie im letzten Jahrhundert. Wiener Medizinische Wochenschrift 39 (1913) 2521–2528; 2521.

[19] STEFAN, J. in "Almanach der kaiserlichen Akademie der Wissenschaften" 29 (1879) 147–172; 153 f.

[20] Eine eingehende Würdigung POLITZERS findet sich bei MAJER, Eduard H.: Adam POLITZER (1835–1920). Laryng. Rhinol. 37 (1978) 769–772.
[21] Trauerfeier für weiland Hofrat POLITZER. Vereinsberichte. Österreichische Otologische Gesellschaft. Sitzung vom 20. Oktober 1920, 57–71; 60.
[22] Das Institut für Geschichte der Medizin der Universität Wien besitzt ein Vortragsmanuskript POLITZERS (HS 582) über Joseph und Arnold TOYNBEE. Dort heißt es: „Wer war Joseph TOYNBEE? Joseph TOYNBEE, zu dem ich das Glück hatte, in freundschaftliche Beziehung zu treten, war der Begründer der pathologischen Anatomie des Gehörorgans, d. h. er war der erste, der eine grosse Anzahl von schwerhörigen Personen untersucht und bei denen er nach dem Tod die Gehörorgane anatomisch zerlegt u. die Ursache der Schwerhörigkeit festgestellt hat. Er hat somit das Fundament der modernen Ohrenheilkunde geschaffen. . . . Die Ergebnisse seiner Forschungen legte er in einem Catalog nieder, welcher die Schilderung von 1659 menschlichen Gehörorganen enthält. . . . Als ich vor 53 Jahren 1861 bei TOYNBEE eingeführt wurde . . ., fand ich bei ihm gastfreundliche Aufnahme. Stundenlang sass er an meiner Seite, um mir die kostbaren Praeparate seiner Sammlung zu erklären. Ich bewahre ihm für die Förderung meiner wissenschaftlichen Laufbahn ein treues Andenken."
[23] Zit. Anm. 10, S. 1327 f.
[24] Zit. Anm. 16, S. 430.
[25] Album, im Besitz des Instituts für Geschichte der Medizin der Universität Wien (U 144). – So meint etwa Theodor BILLROTH im Jahr 1876: „Sehr übel war es bis vor Kurzem um den Unterricht über die Krankheiten des Ohres bestellt. Ich weiss mich aus meiner Studienzeit gut zu erinnern, dass die armen Tauben von einer Klinik in die andere geschickt wurden und Niemand rechte Lust verspürte, sich wirklich für sie zu interessieren. Dies Gebiet ist mit wenigen sehr handgreiflichen Ausnahmen therapeutisch gar zu undankbar. Es ist sehr anerkennenswerth und ein neues Zeichen des unermüdlichen Strebens unserer jetzigen jungen deutschen medicinischen Generation, dass sich nach und nach immer mehr talentvolle Männer finden, welche sich auch in dieses schwierige und undankbare Gebiet vertiefen und es lehren. Klinische otiatrische Ambulatorien gibt es in Berlin, Bern, Halle, Jena, Leipzig, Wien, Zürich; doch so viel ich weiss, besteht nur in Wien eine an zwei Prof. extraordinari vertheilte stationäre Klinik für Ohrenkranke. Es kann nicht davon die Rede sein, solche otiatrische Kliniken für alle Universitäten zu verlangen; dazu würde das Material nicht ausreichen. Mir scheint es opportun, an kleineren Universitäten die Ophthalmologen dazu zu veranlassen, die Otologie mit zu übernehmen, so wenig Neigung sie auch dazu verspüren mögen; wünschenswerth wäre es, dass man dieser kleinen, doch nicht unwichtigen Disciplin irgend einen bestimmten Platz in dem Lehrsystem an den Hochschulen einräumte." (BILLROTH, Th.: Über das Lehren und Lernen der medicinischen Wissenschaften an den Universitäten der Deutschen Nation nebst allgemeinen Bemerkungen über Universitäten. Eine culturhistorische Studie. Wien 1876, S. 123.)
[26] Nekrolog in der Wiener Medizinischen Wochenschrift 50 (1900) 728–730; 729.
[27] Zit. Anm. 26, Sp. 729.
[28] Monatsschrift für Ohrenheilkunde, 1 (1867).

[29] POLITZER, A.: Die Aufgaben des otiatrischen Unterrichtes. Wiener Medicinische Wochenschrift 49 (1899) 325–327; 377–379; 377.

[30] GRUBER, Josef: Lehrbuch der Ohrenheilkunde mit besonderer Rücksicht auf Anatomie und Physiologie. Wien 1870, S. 225. GRUBER beschreibt dort auch das POLITZERsche Verfahren detailliert (S. 226 ff.).

[31] POLITZER, Adam: Lehrbuch der Ohrenheilkunde für practische Ärzte und Studierende. 2 Bde, Stuttgart 1878–1882; Bd. 1, Stuttgart 1878, S. 174: „Da es Jos. GRUBER trotz unablässiger Anstrengungen nicht gelungen, die Anerkennung zu schmälern, welche mein Verfahren in Europa und Amerika gefunden, so hat er später (1870) versucht, für die ihm missliebige Bezeichnung ‚POLITZER'sches Verfahren', die Bezeichnung ‚passiver VALSALVA'scher Versuch' vorzuschlagen und durch die erdichtete, hier wörtlich wiedergegebene Behauptung, (Seite 226 seines Buches) dass schon früher ‚an vielen anderen Stellen und von verschiedenen Autoren auf dieses Manöver aufmerksam gemacht wurde, wenn es auch der grossen Mehrzahl der Nicht-Ohrenärzte unbekannt blieb' glauben zu machen, dass dieses Verfahren schon vor mir in der ohrenärztlichen Literatur bekannt war. In um so grellerem Licht erscheint der obige Vorgang Jos. GRUBER's, der sich nicht scheute, eine LUCAE entlehnte Modifikation des Verschlusses der Gaumenklappe bei meinem Verfahren als eine neue, von ihm erfundene Methode mit grossem Eclat in die Oeffentlichkeit zu bringen, offenbar nur zu dem Zwecke, das von mir angegebene Verfahren, welches er früher als vollkommen überflüssig bezeichnet hat, auf bequeme Weise mit seinem Namen zu belegen. Das ablehnende Verhalten der Fachgenossen und practischen Aerzte konnte indess Prof. Josef GRUBER bald überzeugen, dass diese seine Absicht richtig erkannt und beurtheilt wurde."

[32] Zit. Anm. 16, S. 424.

[33] TRÖLTSCH, F. v.: Das POLITZER'sche Verfahren zur Wegsammachung der Ohrtrompete in seiner Bedeutung für die Ohrenheilkunde. Archiv für die Ohrenheilkunde 1 (1864) 28–43; 43.

[34] Vgl. dazu HOFMANN, L.: Über den Vorläufer des POLITZERschen Verfahrens im Altertum und Mittelalter. Monatsschrift für Ohrenheilkunde und Laryngo-Rhinologie 93 (1959) 330–336.

[35] Statthalterei-Erlaß vom 6. Dezember 1872. Abschrift in der Handschriftensammlung des Instituts für Geschichte der Medizin der Universität Wien, HS 2.093.

[36] Zit. Anm. 35.

[37] Zit. Anm. 16, S. 430.

[38] Zit. Anm. 10, S. 1328.

[39] Zit. Anm. 10, S. 1328.

[40] POLITZER, Adam: Geschichte der Ohrenheilkunde. 2 Bde, Stuttgart 1907–1913, Bd. 2, S. 290.

[41] History of Otology by Dr. Adam POLITZER. Volume I. From earliest times to the middle of the Nineteenth Century. An English translation by Stanley MILSTEIN, Collice PORTNOFF and Antje COLEMAN. Phoenix, Arizona, 1981.

[42] Zit. nach MAJER, E. H., Anm. 20, 772.

[43] STOOL, S. E., B. I. KEMPER and M. J. KEMPER: The Adam POLITZER and Joseph HYRTL Otologic Collections at the Mütter Museum. Transactions & Studies of the College of Physicians of Philadelphia. 4 Ser., Vol. 40, No. 2, Oct. 1972, S. 91–102, S. 93.

[31] POLITZER, Adam: Lehrbuch der Ohrenheilkunde für practische Ärzte und Studierende. 2 vols., Stuttgart, 1878–1882; vol. 1, p. 174: "Since Jos. GRUBER did not succeed – despite continual efforts – in denigrating the reputation which my process enjoys in Europe and America, he later (1870) undertook to suggest as a name for it 'the passive Valsalvan method' instead of 'Politzer's method', which did not suit him. With the following words from his book (page 226) he attempted fallaciously to make us believe that this procedure had already been cited in otological literature: '. . . this maneuver has been mentioned by various authors in many places, even if this fact is not common knowledge among the majority of non-otologists.' GRUBER's behavior appears all the more garish in that he did not shy from publicly declaring that a modification of the closing of the pharynx in my method, which I had adopted from LUCAE, was a newly discovered method of his! Apparently this was only done to be able to conveniently claim as his a method which he had previously maintained to be utterly superfluous. The critical reception which the colleagues of our discipline and the general practitioners have accorded Prof. Josef GRUBER might have convinced him in the meantime that they have recognized and judged his motives correspondingly."

[32] Cited in reference 16, p. 382.

[33] TRÖLTSCH, F. v.: Das POLITZER'sche Verfahren zur Wegsammachung der Ohrtrompete in seiner Bedeutung für die Ohrenheilkunde. Archiv für die Ohrenheilkunde 1 (1864) 28–43; 43.

[34] Cf. HOFMANN, L.: Über den Vorläufer des POLITZERschen Verfahrens im Altertum und Mittelalter. Monatsschrift für Ohrenheilkunde und Laryngo-Rhinologie 93 (1959) 330–336.

[35] Statthalterei-Erlass dated December 6, 1872. Copy in the manuscript collection of the Institute for the History of Medicine of the University of Vienna (HS 2,093).

[36] Cited in reference 35.

[37] Cited in reference 16, p. 388.

[38] Cited in reference 10, p. 1328.

[39] Cited in reference 10, p. 1328.

[40] POLITZER, Adam: Geschichte der Ohrenheilkunde. 2 vols., Stuttgart 1907–1913, vol. 2, p. 290.

[41] History of Otology by Dr. Adam POLITZER. Volume I. From earliest times to the middle of the Nineteenth Century. An English translation by Stanley MILSTEIN, Collice PORTNOFF and Antje COLEMAN. Phoenix, Arizona, 1981.

[42] Cited in reference 20, p. 772.

[43] STOOL, S. E., B. I. KEMPER and M. J. KEMPER: The Adam POLITZER and Joseph HYRTL Otologic Collections at the Mütter Museum. Transactions & Studies of the College of Physicians in Philadelphia. 4 Ser., Vol. 40, No. 2, Oct. 1972, pp. 91–102, p. 93.

[44] Cited in reference 16, p. 389.

[45] Cited in reference 29, 377.

[45a] STOOL, Sylvan E.: A Historical Vignette: Memoirs of an Otologist's European Study in 1883. The American Journal of Otology 4 (1983) 346–349.

[46] Cited in reference 29, 325.

[47] Cited in reference 10, p. 1328.

[48] Cited in reference 20, p. 771.

[49] Cited in reference 10, p. 1329.

[50] Cited in reference 41, p. xiv.

⁴⁴ Zit. Anm. 16, S. 431.
⁴⁵ Zit. Anm. 29, Sp. 377.
⁴⁶ Zit. Anm. 29, Sp. 325.
⁴⁷ Zit. Anm. 10, S. 1328.
⁴⁸ Zit. nach MAJER, E. H., Anm. 20, S. 771.
⁴⁹ Zit. Anm. 10, S. 1329.
⁵⁰ Zit. Anm. 40, Bd. 1, S. V.
⁵¹ Zit. Anm. 16, S. 432.
⁵² Eine ausführliche Darstellung gibt GRÜNEIS, P.: Die Wiener Allgemeine Poliklinik, ihre Entstehung und ihr Werdegang. In: Festschrift zum 80. Geburtstag Max NEUBURGERS. Hrsg. v. E. BERGHOFF, Wien 1948, S. 208–216; und Österr. Ärztezeitung 27 (1972) 667–720.
⁵³ Wiener Medizinische Presse 12 (1871) 1354.
⁵⁴ Ein Ehrentag der allgemeinen Poliklinik. Wiener Medizinische Presse 25 (1884) 1350–1354; 1352.
⁵⁵ Wiener Medizinische Presse 25 (1884) 1352.
⁵⁶ Von der allgemeinen Poliklinik. Wiener Medizinische Presse 13 (1872) 494–495; 494.
⁵⁷ Zit. Anm. 16, S. 337.
⁵⁸ Im Anschluß an den Nachruf von H. NEUMANN in der Monatsschrift für Ohrenheilkunde und Laryngo-Rhinologie 55 (1921) 842–843.
⁵⁹ URBANTSCHITSCH, Viktor: Die Bedeutung der Ohrenheilkunde. Wiener Medizinische Presse 47 (1907). Separatdruck, S. 1 f.
⁶⁰ NEUMANN, H.: Viktor v. URBANTSCHITSCH †. Monatsschrift für Ohrenheilkunde und Laryngo-Rhinologie 55 (1921) 837–842; 839.
⁶¹ Zu ALEXANDER s. den Nachruf von E. URBANTSCHITSCH im Archiv für Ohren-, Nasen- u. Kehlkopfheilkunde Bd. 131, Heft 3 (Sonderdruck) und MAJER, E. H.: Zum 100. Geburtstag von Gustav Alexander und Heinrich Neumann. Österr. Ärztezeitung 29 (1974) 497–500.
⁶² Leider ist dieses Kapitel, wie Erna LESKY, zit. Anm. 16, S. 434, Fußnote 46, schreibt, „vom Menschlichen her belastet". 1916 begannen unerfreuliche Prioritätsstreitigkeiten, weshalb die Verleihung des Professorentitels an BÁRÁNY von der Wiener medizinischen Fakultät abgelehnt wurde. BÁRÁNY nahm daher 1917 eine Berufung nach Uppsala an. Bei einer späteren Einvernahme anläßlich der von BÁRÁNY beantragten Disziplinaruntersuchung erklärten jedoch alle Beteiligten, BÁRÁNY allein gebühre das Verdienst für seine grundlegenden Arbeiten. Vgl. auch DIAMANT, Herman: The Nobel Prize Award for Robert BÁRÁNY – A Controversial Decision? Acta Otolaryngol. (Stockh.) 1984, Suppl. 406, 1–4.
⁶³ Vgl. dazu LESKY, zit. Anm. 16, S. 534 ff.
⁶⁴ Zit. nach MAJER, E. H.: Sonderpostmarke. 100. Geburtstag von Nobelpreisträger Dr. Robert BÁRÁNY, S. 3 f.
⁶⁵ Zu FREMEL s. MAJER, E. H.: Professor Dr. Franz FREMEL zum 75. Geburtstag. Monatsschrift für Ohrenheilkunde und Laryngo-Rhinologie 96 (1962) 327–330 (mit ausführlichem Arbeitenverzeichnis).
⁶⁶ Zit. nach MAJER, E. H., zit. Anm. 64, S. 5 f.
⁶⁷ SCHLANDER, Emil: Die Entwicklung der Ohrenheilkunde an der Wiener Universität. Wiener klinische Wochenschrift 58 (1946) 693–697; 695.
⁶⁸ Wiener klinische Wochenschrift 39 (1926) 16–17; 17.
⁶⁹ ARZT, L.: In memoriam. Wiener klinische Wochenschrift 58 (1946) 117–118; 118.
⁷⁰ Für die Entwicklung in Graz s. insbesondere: MESSERKLIN-

⁵⁰ᵃ LEDERER, Francis L.: A Tribute to Adam Politzer. Archives of Otolaryngology 74 (1961) 130–133; 133.
⁵¹ Cited in reference 16, p. 390.
⁵² A thorough description can be found in GRÜNEIS, P.: Die Wiener Allgemeine Poliklinik, ihre Entstehung und ihr Werdegang. In: Festschrift zum 80. Geburtstag Max NEUBURGERS. Ed. by E. BERGHOFF, Vienna, 1948, pp. 208–216; and Österr. Ärztezeitung 27 (1972) 667–720.
⁵³ Wiener Medizinische Presse 12 (1871) 1354.
⁵⁴ Ein Ehrentag der allgemeinen Poliklinik. Wiener Medizinische Presse 25 (1884) 1350–1354; 1352.
⁵⁵ Wiener Medizinische Presse 25 (1884) 1352.
⁵⁶ Von der allgemeinen Poliklinik. Wiener Medizinische Presse 13 (1872) 494–495; 494.
⁵⁷ Cited in reference 16, p. 301.
⁵⁸ Following the obituary notice by H. NEUMANN in "Monatsschrift für Ohrenheilkunde und Laryngo-Rhinologie" 55 (1921) 842–843.
⁵⁹ URBANTSCHITSCH, Viktor: Die Bedeutung der Ohrenheilkunde. Wiener Medizinische Presse 47 (1907) (reprint, pp. 1 f.)
⁶⁰ NEUMANN, H.: Viktor v. URBANTSCHITSCH. Monatsschrift für Ohrenheilkunde und Laryngo-Rhinologie 55 (1921) 837–842; 839.
⁶¹ For ALEXANDER cf. the obituary notice by E. URBANTSCHITSCH in "Archiv für Ohren-, Nasen- u. Kehlkopfheilkunde", vol. 131, No. 4 (reprint), and MAJER, E. H.: Zum 100. Geburtstag von Gustav ALEXANDER und Heinrich NEUMANN. Österr. Ärztezeitung 29 (1974) 497–500.
⁶² According to E. Lesky (cited in reference 16, p. 392, footnote 46): "This chapter, too, is regrettably influenced by human factors. For the question of priority in regard to the discovery of caloric nystagmus as a diagnostic aid, cf. E. WODAK: Kurze Geschichte der Vestibularisforschung. Stuttgart, 1956, pp. 14 ff.", and DIAMANT, Herman: The Nobel Prize Award for Robert BÁRÁNY – A Controversial Decision? Acta Otolaryngol. (Stockh.) 1984, Suppl. 406, 1–4.
⁶³ Nobel Lecutres including presentation of speeches and laureates' biographies. Physiology or Medicine. 1901–1921. Published for the Nobel Foundation in 1967 by Elsevier Publishing Company, Amsterdam–London–New York, pp. 500–511.
⁶⁴ Cited in reference 63, pp. 500–505.
⁶⁵ For FREMEL cf. MAJER, E. H.: Professor Dr. Franz FREMEL zum 75. Geburtstag. Monatsschrift für Ohrenheilkunde und Laryngo-Rhinologie 96 (1962) 327–330. (With an extensive list of publications.)
⁶⁶ MAJER, E. H.: Sonderpostmarke 100. Geburtstag von Nobelpreisträger Dr. Robert BÁRÁNY, pp. 5 f.
⁶⁷ SCHLANDER, Emil: Die Entwicklung der Ohrenheilkunde an der Wiener Universität. Wiener klinische Wochenschrift 58 (1946) 693–697; 695.
⁶⁸ Wiener klinische Wochenschrift 39 (1926) 16–17; 17.
⁶⁹ ARZT, L.: In memoriam. Wiener klinische Wochenschrift 58 (1946) 117–118; 118.
⁷⁰ For the development in Graz cf. MESSERKLINGER, Walter: Die Leistungen der Grazer Universitätsklinik der Hals-Nasen-Ohrenheilkunde seit ihrer Gründung. Wiener klinische Wochenschrift 72 (1960) 110–113.
⁷¹ Cited in reference 70, p. 111.
⁷² HABERMANN's list of publication can be found in: HOFER,

GER, Walter: Die Leistungen der Grazer Universitätsklinik in der Hals-Nasen-Ohrenheilkunde seit ihrer Gründung. Wiener klinische Wochenschrift 72 (1960) 110–113.

[71] Zit. Anm. 70, S. 111.
[72] Ein ausführliches Arbeitenverzeichnis HABERMANNS findet sich bei: HOFER, Gustav: Johann HABERMANN †. Archiv für Ohren-, Nasen- und Kehlkopfheilkunde. Bd. 139, Heft 4 (Sonderdruck).
[73] Zit. Anm. 3, S. 382.
[74] MOSER, F.: Johannes ZANGE zum 100. Geburtstag. HNO-Praxis 6 (1981) (Sonderdruck).
[75] MESSERKLINGER, W.: Prof. Dr. med. Dr. med. h. c. Gustav HOFER. Monatsschrift für Ohrenheilkunde und Laryngo-Rhinologie 105 (1971) (Sonderdruck).
[76] HÖRBST, L. und W. SCHLORHAUFER: Erinnerungsschrift der Universitätsklinik für Ohren-, Nasen- und Halskrankheiten in Innsbruck anläßlich ihres 60jährigen Bestandes (1893–1953) und ihrer baulichen Erweiterung und Neugestaltung (1953–1956).
[77] HÖRBST, L. und W. SCHLORHAUFER: Klinik für Hals-, Nasen- und Ohrenkrankheiten und Lehrkanzel für Audiologie und Phoniatrie. In: Forschungen zur Innsbrucker Universitätsgeschichte. Hrsg. v. Franz HUTER, VII/2: Hundert Jahre Medizinische Fakultät Innsbruck 1869 bis 1969. 2. Teil Geschichte der Lehrkanzeln, Institute und Kliniken, S. 395–412, S. 411.
[78] SPITZY, K. H. und Inge LAU: Van Swietens Erbe. Die Wiener Medizinische Schule heute in Selbstdarstellungen. Wien–München–Bern 1982, S. 157–164.
[79] SCHRÖTTER, Leopold v.: Festrede, ... Sonderdruck aus „Verhandlungen des I. internationalen Laryngo-Rhinologen-Kongresses", S. 17.
[80] CZERMAK, Johann: Über den Kehlkopfspiegel. Wiener Medizinische Wochenschrift 8 (1858) 196–198.
[81] Zit. Anm. 16, S. 192.
[82] Zit. Anm. 16, S. 192 f.
[83] Zit. Anm. 16, S. 193.
[84] MARSCHIK, Hermann: Geschichte der Wiener laryngo-rhinologischen Gesellschaft im Rahmen der Geschichte der Laryngologie. Wiener klinische Wochenschrift 39 (1926) 334–336; 361–363; 335.
[85] Zit. Anm. 79, S. 23.
[86] Zit. Anm. 16, S. 193.
[87] TÜRCK, L.: Klinik der Krankheiten des Kehlkopfes und der Luftröhre. Wien 1866, Vorrede, S. V.
[88] Darauf hat zum ersten Mal Erna LESKY (zit. Anm. 16, S. 413) hingewiesen.
[89] Zit. Anm. 11, S. 184.
[90] Zit. Anm. 11, S. 184.
[91] Vgl. dazu u. a. IMRE, V.: 100 Jahre Laryngoskopie in Wien. Wiener Medizinische Wochenschrift 108 (1958) 762–764; 763.
[92] MARSCHIK, H.: Festrede zum 100. Geburtstag Leopold v. SCHRÖTTERS. Monatsschrift für Ohrenheilkunde und Laryngo-Rhinologie 71 (1937) 1131–1140; 1134.
[93] Bericht über die 16. Versammlung der Ophthalmologischen Gesellschaft. Heidelberg, 1884. Beilagenheft zu den Klinischen Monatsblättern für Augenheilkunde. XXII. Jg., 60–63; 62 f.
[94] Vgl. dazu und zum folgenden insbes. KOLLER BECKER, Hortense: Carl KOLLER and Cocaine. The Psychoanalytic Quarterly 32 (1963) 309–373; 332 f., und WYKLICKY, H.

Gustav: Johann HABERMANN. Archiv für Ohren-, Nasen- und Kehlkopfheilkunde, vol. 139, nr. 4 (reprint).
[73] Cited in reference 3, p. 382.
[74] MOSER, F.: Johannes ZANGE zum 100. Geburtstag. HNO-Praxis 6 (1981) (reprint).
[75] MESSERKLINGER, W.: Prof. Dr. med. Dr. med. h. c. Gustav HOFER. Monatsschrift für Ohrenheilkunde und Laryngo-Rhinologie 105 (1971) (reprint).
[76] HÖRBST, L. and W. SCHLORHAUFER: Erinnerungsschrift der Universitätsklinik für Ohren-, Nasen- und Halskrankheiten in Innsbruck anläßlich ihres 60jährigen Bestandes (1893–1953) und ihrer baulichen Erweiterung und Neugestaltung (1953–1956).
[77] HÖRBST, L. and W. SCHLORHAUFER: Klinik für Hals-, Nasen- und Ohrenkrankheiten und Lehrkanzel für Audiologie und Phoniatrie. In: Forschungen zur Innsbrucker Universitätsgeschichte. Ed. by Franz HUTER, VII/2: Hundert Jahre Medizinische Fakultät Innsbruck 1869 bis 1969. Part 2: Geschichte der Lehrkanzeln, Institute und Kliniken, pp. 395–412; p. 411.
[78] SPITZY, K. H. and Inge LAU: Van SWIETENS Erbe. Die Wiener Medizinische Schule heute in Selbstdarstellungen. Vienna–Munich–Berne, 1982, pp. 157–164.
[79] SCHRÖTTER, Leopold v.: Festrede, ... Reprint from "Verhandlungen des I. Internationalen Laryngo-Rhinologen-Kongresses" p. 17.
[80] CZERMAK, Johann: Über den Kehlkopfspiegel. Wiener Medizinische Wochenschrift 8 (1858) 196–198.
[81] Cited in reference 16, p. 165.
[82] Cited in reference 16, pp. 165 f.
[83] Cited in reference 16, p. 166.
[84] MARSCHIK, Hermann: Geschichte der Wiener laryngo-rhinologischen Gesellschaft im Rahmen der Geschichte der Laryngologie. Wiener klinische Wochenschrift 39 (1926) 334–336; 361–363; 335.
[85] Cited in reference 79, p. 23.
[86] Cited in reference 16, p. 166.
[87] TÜRCK, L.: Klinik der Krankheiten des Kehlkopfes und der Luftröhre. Vienna, 1866, Vorrede, p. v.
[88] Erna LESKY (cited in reference 16, p. 372) was the first to refer to this fact.
[89] Cited in reference 11, p. 184.
[90] Cited in reference 11, p. 184.
[91] Cf. for instance IMRE, V.: 100 Jahre Laryngoskopie in Wien. Wiener Medizinische Wochenschrift 108 (1958) 762–764; 763.
[92] MARSCHIK, H.: Festrede zum 100. Geburtstag Leopold V. SCHRÖTTERS. Monatsschrift für Ohrenheilkunde und Laryngo-Rhinologie 71 (1937) 1131–1140; 1134.
[93] Bericht über die 16. Versammlung der Ophthalmologischen Gesellschaft. Heidelberg, 1884. Beilagenheft zu den Klinischen Monatsblättern für Augenheilkunde. XXII. Jg., 60–63; 62 f.
[94] Cf. for this and the following especially KOLLER BECKER, Hortense: Carl KOLLER and Cocaine. The Psychoanalytic Quarterly 32 (1963) 309–373; 332 f., and WYCKLICKY, H. and M. SKOPEC: Carl KOLLER (1857–1944) and His Time in Vienna. In: Regional Anaesthesia 1884–1984. Ed. by D. B. SCOTT, J. Mc CLURE, J. A. W. WILDSMITH. Södertälje, Sweden, 1984, pp. 12–16.
[95] FREUD, S.: Beitrag zur Kenntnis der Cocawirkung. Wiener Medizinische Wochenschrift 35 (1885) 129–133; 129.

und M. Skopec: Carl Koller (1857–1944) and His Time in Vienna. In: Regional Anaesthesia 1884–1984. Ed. by D. B. Scott, J. McClure, J. A. W. Wildsmith. Södertälje, Sweden, 1984, S. 12–16.

⁹⁵ Freud, S.: Beitrag zur Kenntnis der Cocawirkung. Wiener Medizinische Wochenschrift 35 (1885) 129–133; 129.

⁹⁶ Koller, Carl: Nachträgliche Bemerkungen über die ersten Anfänge der Lokalanästhesie. Wiener Medizinische Wochenschrift 85 (1935) 7–8.

⁹⁷ Medizinische Jahrbücher der k. k. Gesellschaft der Ärzte 1885. Anzeiger Nr. 2, S. 11.

⁹⁸ Jelinek, E.: Das Cocain als Anästheticum und Analgeticum für den Pharynx und Larynx. Wiener Medizinische Wochenschrift 34 (1884) 1334–1337, 1364–1367.

⁹⁹ Sorgo, J.: Über die Behandlung der Kehlkopftuberkulose mit reflektiertem Sonnenlichte. (Vorläufige Mitteilung.) Wiener klinische Wochenschrift 17 (1904) 12–14; Sorgo, J.: Über die Behandlung der Kehlkopftuberkulose mit Sonnenlicht nebst einem Vorschlag zur Behandlung derselben mit künstlichem Licht. Wiener klinische Wochenschrift 18 (1905) 87–89; Sorgo, J.: Methodik und Behandlung der Lungentuberkulose mit Sonnenlicht und künstlichem Licht. Wiener Medizinische Wochenschrift 71 (1921) 2206–2210.

¹⁰⁰ Sattler, A.: Univ.-Prof. Dr. Josef Sorgo – 80 Jahre alt. Österr. Ärztezeitung 5 (1949) 40.

¹⁰¹ Lebenserinnerungen des Hermann Arthur Thost, geboren 9. Juni 1854, gestorben 23. Dezember 1937. Typoskript im Besitz von E. H. Majer, S. 51.

¹⁰² Zit. Anm. 16, S. 414.

¹⁰³ Chiari, O.: Karl Stoerk. Wiener klinische Wochenschrift 12 (1899) 954–955; 955.

¹⁰⁴ Zit. Anm. 16, S. 406 f.

¹⁰⁵ Prof. Stoerk †. Wiener Medizinische Wochenschrift 49 (1899) 1772–1773; 1772.

¹⁰⁶ Zit. Anm. 16, S. 407.

¹⁰⁷ Zitiert nach Lesky, E., zit. Anm. 16, S. 408.

¹⁰⁸ Zit. Anm. 16, S. 409.

¹⁰⁹ Zit. Anm. 16, S. 410.

¹¹⁰ Zit. Anm. 105, Sp. 1773.

¹¹¹ Zit. Anm. 16, S. 412.

¹¹² Zit. Anm. 16, S. 418.

¹¹³ Vgl. dazu Worbs, Michael: Nervenkunst. Literatur und Psychoanalyse im Wien der Jahrhundertwende. Frankfurt a. Main 1983.

¹¹⁴ Internationale Rundschau, Jg. 1889 (Sonderdruck).

¹¹⁵ Vgl. dazu Speck, Reiner: Die Allgemeine Wiener Poliklinik und „Professor Bernhardi". Zum hospitalhistorischen und biographischen Hintergrund in Arthur Schnitzlers gleichnamiger Komödie. In: Historia Hospitalium, Heft 14, 1981/82, S. 301–320, und Kindlers Literaturlexikon, Bd. IX, Darmstadt 1972, S. 7810.

¹¹⁶ Marschik, Hermann: Zur Geschichte der Laryngo-Rhinologie an der Wiener Allgemeinen Poliklinik. Wiener Medizinische Wochenschrift 78 (1928) 1579–1581; 79 (1929) 1511–1516, 1587–1590.

¹¹⁷ Gussenbauer, Carl: Über die erste durch Th. Billroth am Menschen ausgeführte Kehlkopf-Exstirpation und die Anwendung eines künstlichen Kehlkopfes. Langenbeck's Archiv für klinische Chirurgie 17 (1874) 343–356.

¹¹⁸ Vgl. dazu auch Majer, E. H.: 100 Jahre Kehlkopfexstirpation. Laryngologie, Rhinologie, Otologie 54 (1975) 3–9,

⁹⁶ Koller, Carl: Nachträgliche Bemerkungen über die ersten Anfänge der Lokalanästhesie. Wiener Medizinische Wochenschrift 85 (1935) 7–8.

⁹⁷ Medizinische Jahrbücher der k. k. Gesellschaft der Ärzte 1885. Anzeiger Nr. 2, p. 11.

⁹⁸ Jelinek, E.: Das Cocain als Anästheticum und Analgeticum für den Pharynx und Larynx. Wiener Medizinische Wochenschrift 34 (1884) 1334–1337, 1364–1367.

⁹⁹ Sorgo, J.: Über die Behandlung der Kehlkopftuberkulose mit reflektiertem Sonnenlichte. (Vorläufige Mitteilung.) Wiener klinische Wochenschrift 17 (1904) 12–14; Sorgo, J.: Über die Behandlung der Kehlkopftuberkulose mit Sonnenlicht nebst einem Vorschlag zur Behandlung derselben mit künstlichem Licht. Wiener klinische Wochenschrift 18 (1905) 87–89; Sorgo, J.: Methodik und Behandlung der Lungentuberkulose mit Sonnenlicht und künstlichem Licht. Wiener Medizinische Wochenschrift 71 (1921) 2206–2210.

¹⁰⁰ Sattler, A.: Univ.-Prof. Dr. Josef Sorgo – 80 Jahre alt. Österr. Ärztezeitung 5 (1949) 40.

¹⁰¹ Lebenserinnerungen des Hermann Arthur Thost, geboren 9. Juni 1854, gestorben 23. Dezember 1937. Typoscript in the possession of E. H. Majer, p. 51.

¹⁰² Cited in reference 16, p. 373.

¹⁰³ Chiari, O.: Karl Stoerk. Wiener klinische Wochenschrift 12 (1899) 954–955; 955.

¹⁰⁴ Cited in reference 16, p. 366.

¹⁰⁵ Prof. Stoerk †. Wiener Medizinische Wochenschrift 49 (1899) 1772–1773; 1772.

¹⁰⁶ Cited in reference 16, pp. 366 f.

¹⁰⁷ Cited in reference 16, p. 367.

¹⁰⁸ Cited in reference 16, pp. 368 f.

¹⁰⁹ Cited in reference 16, p. 369.

¹¹⁰ Cited in reference 105, 1773.

¹¹¹ Cited in reference 16, pp. 371 f.

¹¹² Cited in reference 16, p. 376.

¹¹³ Cf. Worbs, Michael: Nervenkunst. Literatur und Psychoanalyse im Wien der Jahrhundertwende. Frankfurt a. Main, 1983.

¹¹⁴ Internationale Rundschau, Jg. 1889 (reprint).

¹¹⁵ Cf. Speck, Reiner: Die Allgemeine Wiener Poliklinik und "Professor Bernhardi". Zum hospitalhistorischen und biographischen Hintergrund in Arthur Schnitzlers gleichnamiger Komödie. In: Historia Hospitalium, Heft 14, 1981/82, pp. 301–320, and Kindlers Literaturlexikon, vol. IX, Darmstadt, 1972, p. 7810.

¹¹⁶ Marschik, Hermann: Zur Geschichte der Laryngo-Rhinologie an der Wiener Allgemeinen Poliklinik. Wiener Medizinische Wochenschrift 78 (1928) 1579–1581; 79 (1929) 1511–1516, 1587–1590.

¹¹⁷ Gussenbauer, Carl: Über die erste durch Th. Billroth am Menschen ausgeführte Kehlkopf-Exstirpation und die Anwendung eines künstlichen Kehlkopfes. Langenbeck's Archiv für klinische Chirurgie 17 (1874) 343–356.

¹¹⁸ Absolon, Karel B.: First Laryngectomy for Cancer as Performed by Theodor Billroth on December 31, 1873: A Hundred Anniversary. Review of Surgery, vol. 31, no. 2 (1974) 65–70.

¹¹⁹ Cited in reference 11, p. 188.

¹²⁰ Majer, E. H.: Die Hals-Nasen-Ohren-Abteilung. Österr. Ärztezeitung 27 (1972) 693–699; 695.

¹²¹ Cf. Wyklicky, Helmut: Musikalische Ärzte am Anfang

[119] Zit. Anm. 11, S. 188.
[120] MAJER, E. H.: Die Hals-Nasen-Ohren-Abteilung. Österr. Ärztezeitung 27 (1972) 693–699; 695.
[121] Vgl. dazu insbesondere WYKLICKY, Helmut: Musikalische Ärzte am Anfang unseres Jahrhunderts. Österr. Ärztezeitung. Sammlung der Titelblätter des Jahres 1975, Nr. 23.
[122] Zit. Anm. 11, S. 188.
[123] WYKLICKY, Helmut: Der Vater der endonasalen Chirurgie. Österr. Ärztezeitung. Sammlung der Titelblätter des Jahres 1975, Nr. 15/16.
[124] MAJER, E. H.: Zur Geschichte der HNO-Heilkunde in Österreich. Laryng. Rhinol. 59 (1980) 406–411; 410.
[125] HOFER, Gustav: Herrn Professor Dr. M. HAJEK zum 70. Geburtstage. Wiener Medizinische Wochenschrift 81 (1931) 1547–1548.
[126] WIETHE, Camillo: Dem Andenken Markus HAJEKs. Monatsschrift für Ohrenheilkunde 7 (1946) (Separatdruck).
[127] Zit. Anm. 11, S. 187.
[128] Zu KAFKAS letzten Lebensjahren s. die ausgezeichnete Monographie von HACKERMÜLLER, Rotraut: Das Leben, das mich stört. Wien–Berlin 1984.
[129] Zit. Anm. 128, S. 106.
[130] Zit. Anm. 128, S. 124.
[131] Vgl. dazu auch RODEGRA, H.: Die Anfänge der Endoskopie. Laryng. Rhinol. 58 (1979) 723–730.
[132] WESSELY baute die Behandlung der Schleimhauttuberkulose mit künstlichem Sonnenlicht auf und richtete wegen der damals häufigen Kehlkopftuberkulose eine eigene Tuberkulose-Ambulanz an der Klinik ein. Er verbesserte auch die Technik der Totalexstirpation bei Kehlkopftumoren und vereinfachte die Nachbehandlung. Vgl. dazu MAJER, E. H., zit. Anm. 124, S. 411.
[133] Zit. Anm. 78, S. 154.

und WYKLICKY, Helmut: Vor hundert Jahren.... Wiener Medizinische Wochenschrift 131 (1981) 1–13.

unseres Jahrhunderts. Österr. Ärztezeitung. Sammlung der Titelblätter des Jahres 1975, nr. 23.
[122] Cited in reference 11, p. 188.
[123] WYKLICKY, Helmut: Der Vater der endonasalen Chirurgie. Österr. Ärztezeitung. Sammlung der Titelblätter des Jahres 1975, Nr. 15/16.
[124] MAJER, E. H.: Zur Geschichte der HNO-Heilkunde in Österreich. Laryng. Rhinol. 59 (1980) 406–411; 410.
[125] HOFER, Gustav: Herrn Professor Dr. M. HAJEK zum 70. Geburtstage. Wiener Medizinische Wochenschrift 81 (1931) 1547–1548.
[126] WIETHE, Camillo: Dem Andenken Markus HAJEKs. Monatsschrift für Ohrenheilkunde 7 (1946) (reprint).
[127] Cited in reference 11, p. 187.
[128] Refer to the last years of KAFKA's life in the excellent monograph: HACKERMÜLLER, Rotraut: Das Leben, das mich stört. Vienna–Berlin, 1984.
[129] Cited in reference 128, p. 106.
[130] Cited in reference 128, p. 124.
[131] Cf. RODEGRA, H.: Die Anfänge der Endoskopie. Laryng. Rhinol. 58 (1979) 723–730.
[132] WESSELY established the treatment for tuberculosis of the mucosa using artifical sunlight and founded an out-patient clinic for the treatment of tuberculosis of the larynx, which occurred frequently at that time. He also improved upon the technique for radical laryngectomies.
[133] Cited in reference 78, p. 154.

DIE VORSTÄNDE DER UNIVERSITÄTSKLINIKEN IN
WIEN, GRAZ UND INNSBRUCK.
DIE ABTEILUNGSVORSTÄNDE DER ALLGEMEINEN POLIKLINIK IN WIEN.

Zusammengestellt von Eduard H. MAJER

THE HEADS OF THE UNIVERSITY CLINICS
IN VIENNA, GRAZ AND INNSBRUCK.
THE HEADS OF DEPARTMENTS OF THE GENERAL POLICLINIC IN VIENNA.

Compiled by Eduard H. MAJER

UNIVERSITÄTSOHRENKLINIK, WIEN

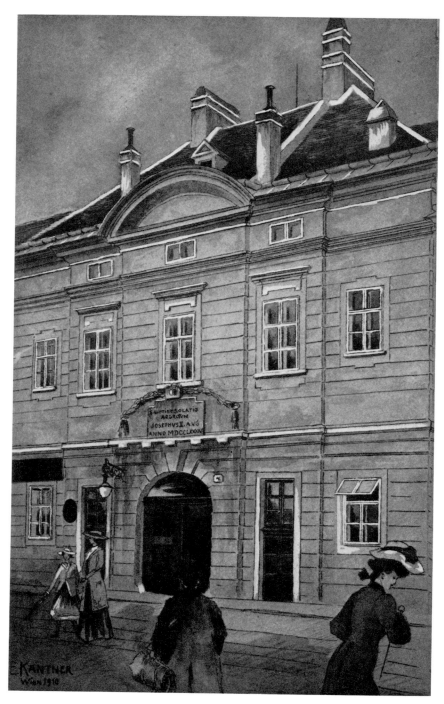

Haupteingang zum Wiener Allgemeinen Krankenhaus.
Aquarell von E. Kantner, Wien 1910.

*Main entrance to the Vienna General Hospital.
Watercolor by E. Kantner, Vienna, 1910.*

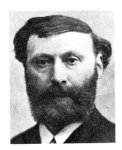
ADAM POLITZER
1873–1907

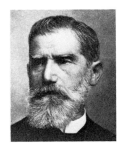
JOSEF GRUBER
1873–1898

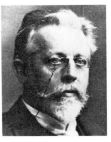
VIKTOR VON
URBANTSCHITSCH
1907–1918

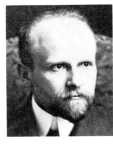
ROBERT BÁRÁNY
Nobelpreis 1914

Klinik für Ohren-, Nasen-,
Kehlkopfkrankheiten

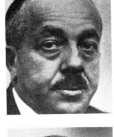
HEINRICH NEUMANN
1919–1938

Ab 1938
I. Univ. Hals-, Nasen-, Ohrenklinik

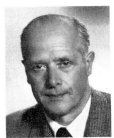
SIEGFRIED UNTERBERGER
1939–1945

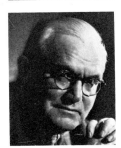
EMIL SCHLANDER
1945–1959

1963–1969
Filialstation der II. HNO-Klinik

Ab 1970
II. HNO-Klinik

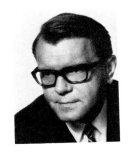
KURT BURIAN
bis 1969

1970–

LARYNGOLOGISCHE UNIVERSITÄTSKLINIK, WIEN

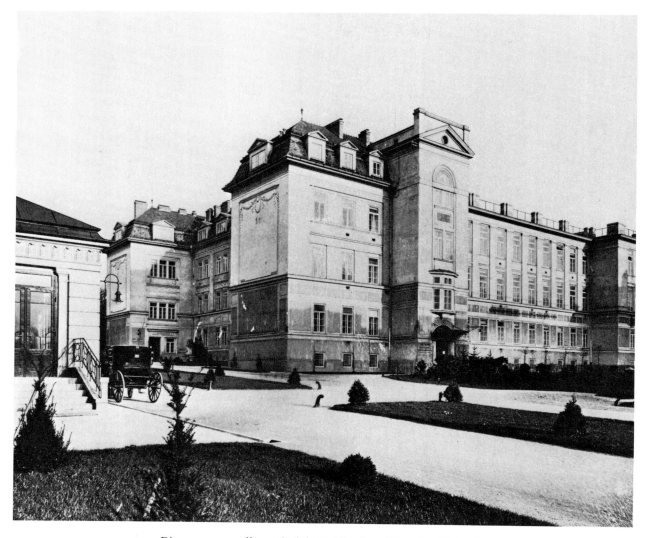

Die neue, 1911 eröffnete Klinik für Kehlkopf- und Nasenkrankheiten in Wien IX, Lazarettgasse 14.

The new Clinic for Diseases of the Larynx and the Nose, which was opened in Vienna's ninth district, Lazarettgasse 14, in 1911.

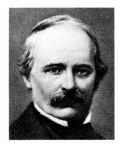
Ludwig Türck

1870 Gründung der Klinik

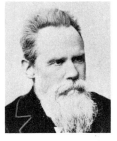
Leopold Schrötter von Kristelli
1870–1890

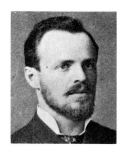
E. Jelinek,
Assistent der Klinik
1884: Kokain zur Kehlkopf-Anästhesie

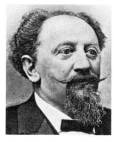
Karl Stoerk
1890–1899

1911 Eröffnung
der neuen Klinik f. Kehlkopf- und Nasenkrankheiten

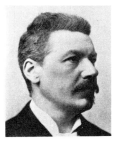
Ottokar von Chiari
1899–1918

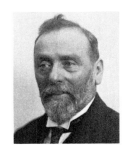
Markus Hajek
1919–1933

Laryngologische Station
der Univ. Ohrenklinik
II. Univ. HNO-Klinik
1938–1969

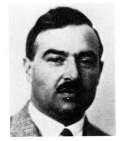
Emil Wessely
1934–1938

Emil Wessely
1953–1954

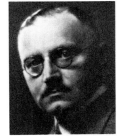
Camillo Wiethe
1945–1949

Ab 1970:
I. Univ. HNO-Klinik

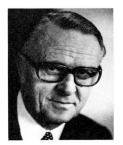
Otto Novotny
1955–1982

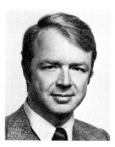
Klaus Ehrenberger
1983–

UNIVERSITÄTSKLINIK FÜR OHREN-, NASEN-, HALSKRANKHEITEN, GRAZ

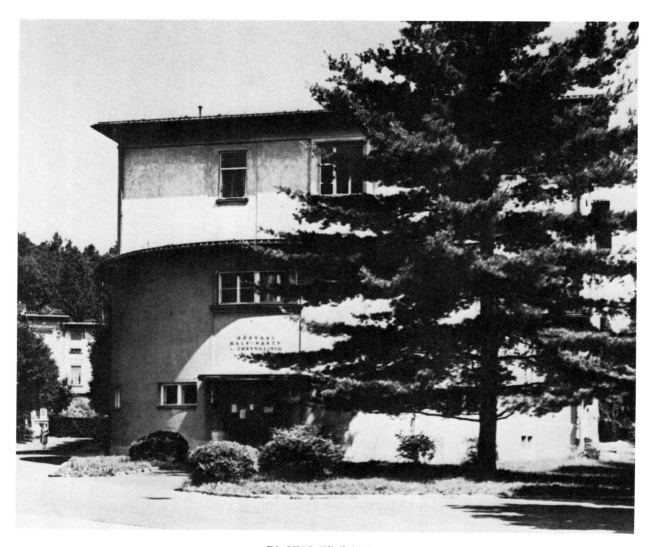

Die HNO-Klinik in Graz.
The ENT-Clinic in Graz.

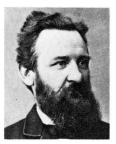
Johann Kessel
1875 1. Stapesmobilisation

1893 Eröffnung der Klinik

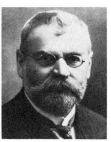
Johann Habermann
1893–1922

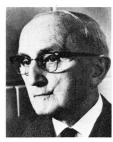
Johannes Zange
1922–1931

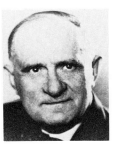
Gustav Hofer
1931–1959

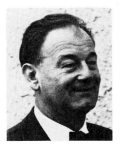
Walter Messerklinger
1959–

UNIVERSITÄTSKLINIK FÜR HALS-, NASEN-, OHRENKRANKHEITEN, INNSBRUCK

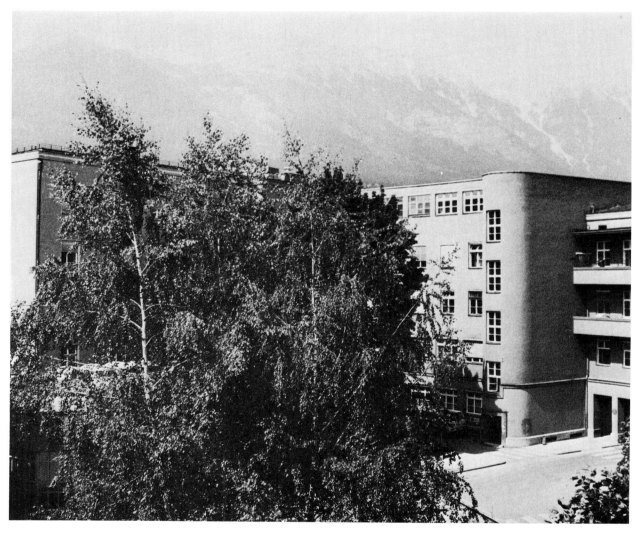

Die HNO-Klinik in Innsbruck

The ENT-Clinic in Innsbruck.

1894 Eröffnung der Klinik

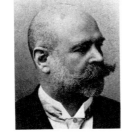

Georg Juffinger
1893–1913

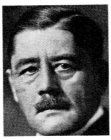

Heinrich Herzog
1916–1928

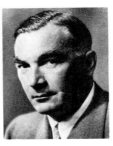

Wilfried Krainz
1928–1943

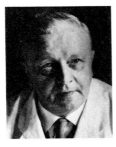

Werner Kindler
1944–1945

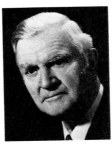

Ludwig Hörbst
1945–1974

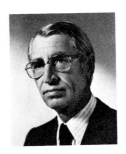

Walter Schlorhaufer
1968 Lehrkanzel f. Audiologie u. Phoniatrie

1974 Univ.-Klinik f. Hör-, Sprach- und Stimmstörungen

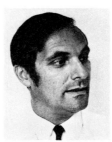

Heinrich Spoendlin
1976–

ALLGEMEINE POLIKLINIK, WIEN

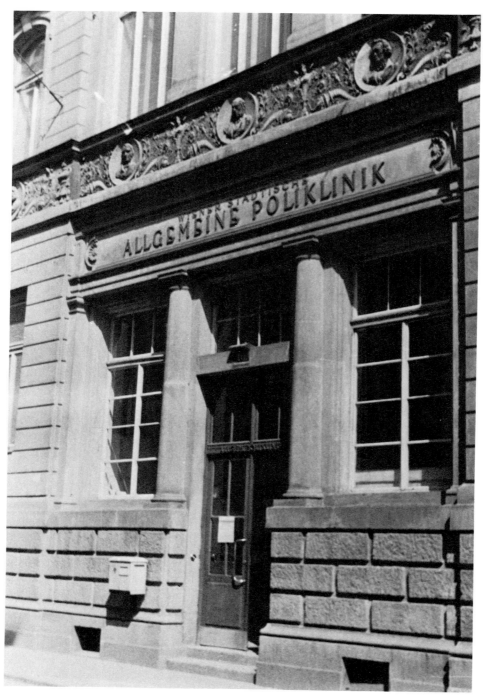

Haupteingang zur Poliklinik nach der Restaurierung.

Main entrance to the Vienna General Policlinic after its restoration.

OTOLOGIE

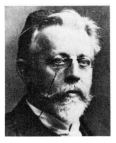

Viktor von
Urbanitschitsch
1872–1907

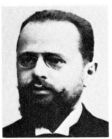

Gustav Alexander
1907–1932

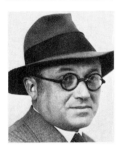

Hans Brunner
1932–1938

LARYNGOLOGIE

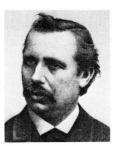

Johann Schnitzler
1871–1893

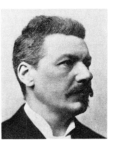

Ottokar von
Chiari
1893–1899

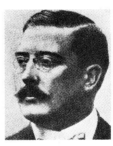

Hans Koschier
1900–1918

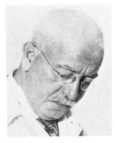

Hermann Marschik
H.N.: 1920–1938
H.N.O.: –1946

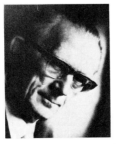

Eduard H. Majer
H.N.O. 1946–1974

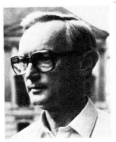

Ernst Moritsch
H.N.O. 1974–